LINDA MACCRACKEN

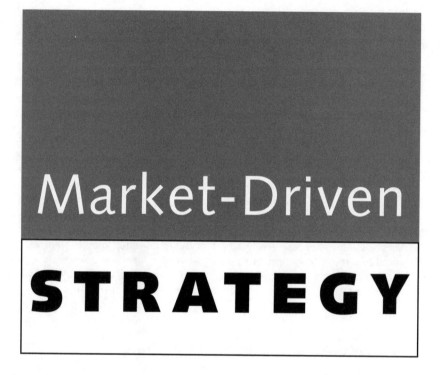

Market-Driven

STRATEGY

An Executive Guide to Health Care's Integrated Environment

This publication is designed to provide accurate and authoritative information in regard to the subject matter covered. It is sold with the understanding that neither the author nor the publisher is engaged in rendering legal, accounting, or other professional service. If legal advice or other expert assistance is required, the services of a competent professional should be sought.

The views expressed in this publication are strictly those of the authors and do not necessarily represent official positions of the American Hospital Association.

Cover design by Andrea Federle-Bucsi

Library of Congress Cataloging-in-Publication Data

MacCracken, Linda.
    Market-driven strategy : an executive's guide to
health care's integrated environment / by Linda
MacCracken
    p.   cm.
    Includes index.
1. Health planning—Economic aspects I. Title.
RA410.5.M25 1998
362.1'068'4—dc21

97-28826
CIP

ISBN: 1-55648-211-6

Item Number: 127152

For Jim and Sarah

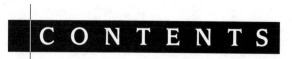

CONTENTS

About the Author   *vii*

Preface   *ix*

Acknowledgments   *xiii*

CHAPTER 1   **Trends in Health Care Delivery Planning**   1
Current State of Health Care Delivery   2
Planning as a Tool for Being Prepared   3
Integrating the Organization's Strategic Directions
    into a Strategic Plan   6
Planning's Role in the Development of
    Health Care Service Delivery   12
Merging Roles of Payers and Providers   25
Conclusion   29

CHAPTER 2   **The Strategic Plan Development Process**   33
Steps in the Process of Strategic Plan Development   34
Past Problems with Strategic Plan Development   62
Conclusion   66

CHAPTER 3   **Assessment of the Environment**   69
Identifying Industry Drivers   70
The Payer/Provider Landscape   75
Models for Performing an Industry Analysis   78
Frameworks for Assessing the Health Care Industry   85
Approach to Affiliation   104
Lessons Learned from Performing
    Environmental Analyses   106
Conclusion   108

CHAPTER 4   **The Approach to Strategic Plan
Implementation**   111
Articulation   112
Activation   119

	Ability	123
	Past Problems with Strategic Plan Implementation	128
	Conclusion	132
CHAPTER 5	**Action Steps in Strategic Plan Implementation**	135
	Components of the Implementation Process	136
	Moving toward Managed Care and Integration	143
	Collaborative Marketing	167
	Conclusion	180
CHAPTER 6	**Strategy as a Part of Organizational Life**	183
	Strategic Plan Review and Update	184
	Conclusion	204
	Index	207

ABOUT THE AUTHOR

Linda MacCracken has more than 15 years of experience in health care planning and marketing. She has worked in, and with, academic, managed care, and community-based organizations in Minneapolis and Boston (including executive-level positions at Boston's Beth Israel Hospital and other community hospitals). A graduate-level instructor, she has taught health care marketing courses at the Harvard School of Public Health, the Graduate School of Management at Boston University, and Northeastern University's Graduate School of Management. Ms. MacCracken is a frequent presenter to the AHA Society for Healthcare Planning and Marketing, the American Marketing Association, and the Healthcare Strategy Institute. Her topics range from strategic and marketing planning to marketing-to-win. She is currently chief market planning officer and vice president of market services at Sturdy Memorial Hospital in eastern Massachusetts. She earned her B.A. in psychology from Macalester College in Minnesota and her M.B.A. in health care management from Boston University.

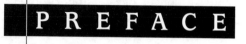

PREFACE

Market-Driven Strategy: An Executive's Guide to Health Care's Integrated Environment is about how to develop and implement strategy in health care organizations. It reviews trends in health care strategy and assesses effective models and practices for strategy development and implementation. It also details the activities and processes that organizations can use to transform environmental confusion into a purposeful future, harnessing the contribution of the many capable people participating in and outside the organization. Because health care delivery is a local business—whether providers are consolidated locally or on a larger geographic area—the strategic issues are directed by the local market considerations. Therefore, regardless of the consolidation structure, this book reviews local and regional factors and its response for the health care provider.

BACKGROUND

Traditionally, health care planning has followed a course of maximizing services and reimbursement according to available resources. The post–World War II era supported facility development, provided for unconstrained growth in health care, and, consequently, offered providers little incentive to manage health care costs. And despite the onset of utilization review, there were few incentives to manage overall quality. But now, the advent of competition with a free-market orientation and the change from cost-based reimbursement to case-mix reimbursement (managed care) has led to a search for processes that will foster quality and overall health management.

Health care delivery system drivers are changing at a radical pace, in concert with changing public and private financing mechanisms and public perceptions. Payment trends no longer dictate strategic directions, because they change rapidly and there are other drivers shaping these trends that have greater implications for the future of the delivery system.

The customer is king. This theme is the only stable component of the health care delivery system, as service purchase decisions are increasingly user-driven. This is in sharp contrast to prior years, when the customer was the helpless bystander in the system.

The health care delivery system responds to the structure of regional health care delivery markets, despite the presence of national players and uniform payment proposals from a variety of reform initiatives. Therefore, the shape of the marketplace drives the strategy formation, requiring that organizations assess the scope of the market in which they operate.

ROLE OF STRATEGIC PLANNING

Strategic planning has historically relied on that which is known. While the past is only effective as a guidepost, it is often mistaken for a hitching post. Organizations chart their future direction based on what they know without incorporating what they are willing to believe. Most notably, the failures of strategy are attributable to many factors, including (1) lack of management commitment, (2) lack of employee alignment, and (3) cumbersome planning processes without an overarching vision. Strategic plan development only works with a management commitment to support development, to align employees, and to flexibly implement the strategic plan.

Strategic plan development charts the organization's future. As active parts of the management agenda, the strategy components rely on a vision statement that reflects both the expected and the desired futures. On a practical basis, strategy decisions are based on six factors:

- Payer assessment and position
- Physician network assessment and position
- Organizational and financial capabilities and performance
- Merger and alliance positions
- Getting and keeping groups of customers
- Action plan development

AUDIENCE

Market-Driven Strategy is written for executives, managers, and professionals who are interested in or working on charting the future of their health care organization. Those who formulate strategy and engage others to participate in its implementation work within a unique set of partnerships, and it is toward this group that the book is targeted. Such partnerships are shared by executives, clinical managers, physician executives, and other active participants in the strategic management of the health care organization.

OVERVIEW

Chapter 1, "Trends in Health Care Delivery Planning," presents an overview of patterns in strategic plan development. Most planning actions have traditionally mirrored trends in reimbursement and market conditions. The merging roles of payers, acute care providers, and physicians, which demonstrate varying degrees of integration and marketplace consolidation, now must be taken into consideration in any planning process. This chapter also discusses the attention given to payers and primary care providers by health care systems as a new means of securing business.

The components of a strategic plan development process and the implications for its implementation are the focus of chapter 2, "The Strategic Plan Development Process." Problems and difficulties of strategic plan development include lack of commitment and employee alignment, inflexible systems, and cumbersome planning processes. Effective strategy development relies on vision, values, environmental analysis, and practical alliances. The chapter discusses the pitfalls of strategic plan development and reviews the components of a strategy platform.

Chapter 3, "Assessment of the Environment," reviews the components necessary to conduct an environmental assessment. The process starts with a scan of business drivers for strategic change and an analysis of their relevance to health care. The chapter presents frameworks for assessing national trends, regional trends, and local trends, as well as approaches to looking at potential local, regional, and national alliance partners.

The three principles required for effective strategy implementation are presented in chapter 4, "The Approach to Strategic Plan Implementation." They are

- *Articulation:* using vision and values in interaction with the employees to align them with the strategic directions
- *Activation:* completing the action steps of the strategic plan while allowing for flexibility
- *Ability:* ensuring the proper skill and experience to perform the new activities of the organization

The chapter also discusses the problems and difficulties of strategic plan implementation, including lack of organizational alignment, failure to measure expected and actual impact, and other transition problems.

Chapter 5, "Action Steps in Strategic Plan Implementation," reviews the components of implementation. These include the processes of designating accountability for the initiatives, focusing management attention on the implementation, and making the requisite updates and revisions while accounting for actual and expected results. The chapter presents activities organizations must engage in to achieve and incorporate a vision. Examples of organizations experiencing progressive change toward integration, responding to and preparing for greater levels of managed care, and developing new approaches to collaborative marketing and relationship marketing are analyzed. Contingencies and the resolution of new challenges found during implementation are also discussed.

The book closes with a review of the activities involved in organizational life in the period between planning cycles, in chapter 6, "Strategy as a Part of Organizational Life." Such activities include establishing varying degrees of integration, working with payers, and responding to customers based on community needs. Strategic monitoring and providing relevant updates to the plan can both complete one implementation and prepare for the next strategy development. With new alliances and a new organization, the relationships with constituents and the strategic directions may need to be adjusted. The chapter mentions the new priorities and problems that often arise as a result of the implemented initiatives.

ACKNOWLEDGMENTS

I am grateful to the many people who gave generously of their time to discuss the issues in this book, especially Laura Avakian, Russ Coile, Nancy Dubler, Carolyn Jacobi Gabbay, Paul Gleichauf, David Kantor, George Koller, Jeffrey J. Lefko, David Lincoln, James MacCracken, Virginia Manzella, David Marlowe, Mark Mazak, Rosemary Mathias, Greg Nelson, Philip Newbold, Peter Rabinowitz, Jane Saks, Dr. Richard Shea, Dr. Louise Schneider, Douglas Spencer, and Rhoda Weiss. I wish to acknowledge the indispensable work of my research assistant, Danielle Celona, whose research over several years was instrumental.

I wish to thank all my professors, especially Lloyd Baird, Roberta N. Clarke, Charles Green, James Post, and Theodore Murray, for teaching me about strategy. Special thanks to Dr. Mitchell T. Rabkin for encouraging me to write a book in the first place. I also thank Lauren Barnett and the Society for Healthcare Strategy and Market Development for their support of this project and for stimulating educational programs that have greatly contributed to this book. I'm indebted to my colleagues, by whom I have been immeasurably challenged and from whom I have learned a great deal about strategic success.

I owe special thanks to Judy Neiman, who got this project started and has continued to offer extraordinary support; and to Donna Soodalter-Toman, for long discussions and insights about strategic issues.

I thank Mark Swartz, project editor at AHPI, for the skillful job he did in finalizing the manuscript, and I appreciate the efforts of all the staff. I owe a special debt to Richard Hill, senior editor. He has always been there when I needed him.

And finally, I reserve my deepest thanks to my husband, Jim Champlin, who sustained me throughout this enterprise.

Trends in Health Care Delivery Planning

It was the best of times, it was the worst of times.

—*Charles Dickens*

Executive Summary

Health care delivery has changed recently, partly because of the policies that support its funding and growth and partly because of the emergence of private companies that appeal to specific customer groups. Principally founded in a not-for-profit market, health care institutions have flourished through the social commitment—funded by government programs—to increase access, and through the patronage of communities sponsoring their own local health care providers.

Historically, health care planning has followed a course of maximizing services and reimbursement according to available resources and market conditions. The post–World War II boom supported facility development. The 1960s saw the onset of cost-based reimbursement from Medicare and Medicaid. And the 1980s and 1990s brought the rise of competitive pressures, diversification, and the growth of managed care. Managed care penetration and provider consolidation are both different, and health care delivery is more regional now than when federal government parameters shaped the industry.

INTRODUCTION

Planning is charting, continually evaluating the future of, and redirecting an organization to assure the means of obtaining resources to achieve desired outcomes, and to assure that those outcomes align with market desires. It started as, and continues to be, a practice meant to obtain more resources through the regulatory channels to serve the community. Additionally, planning is a way to develop a competitive edge by taking advantage of available resources. For example, planning is required to take advantage of federal programs that pay for facility development, and to form a strategic assessment of the market in order to obtain capital through debt financing or stock offerings.

While managed care is a factor in the drive to the integration of health care delivery, so is securing customers through traditional channels (large payer groups, Medicare, and Medicaid) and nontraditional channels (healthier individual and illness prevention initiatives). Directing an organization's business and market position is still the core of the planning activity. With the shift of Medicare and Medicaid to prepaid managed care programs, interest is rising in capitation, total community health, and long-term health management. An integrated delivery system is a combination of both inpatient and outpatient care modalities in one organizational entity. More specifically, it is defined as "an economic and operational concept where various components of the health care delivery system have the same interests and objectives."[1] Employers' increasingly active direction is also taking hold. Competitive pressures to do more with fewer resources and to consolidate a fragmented delivery system vary among different markets, yet they push all health care providers to view themselves and their world differently.

The market-specific characteristics and frequent public attention to both the business changes (with provider consolidation) and the clinical issues (with publicity for quality errors) raise the public's concern about both the business focus and the clinical quality of health care. Health care organizations are responding by focusing on consumers, taking more polls and employing more sophisticated satisfaction systems and more nontraditional ways to reach out to customers.

This chapter reviews major trends in health care delivery planning and highlights the merging roles of payers, acute care providers, and physicians. The chapter also describes the health care system's attention to payers and primary care providers as a means of securing business.

CURRENT STATE OF HEALTH CARE DELIVERY

Health care delivery is in a state of flux. Now more than ever, this government-sponsored industry has been shedding its regulatory support and constraints and creating more incentives to move health care to the private sector. Providers continue to support the deregulated industry, while policy makers continue to advocate services for all persons through private means. Capitation, the anticipated means of payment expected in some form of payer reform (certainly in Medicare and

Medicaid, and, increasingly, from large employers), has precipitated a move by many toward integrated delivery systems (IDSs) or integrated delivery and financing systems (IDFS). In this flux, however, some health care providers have moved to become IDSs, some are in the midst of negotiations to become integrated, and others are divesting portions of the businesses that would make them IDSs.

The health care industry is a focus of change and ongoing complaints. Employers say their premiums are increasing with unclear cause. Consumers believe that health care consumes too much of the gross national product (GNP) over the past four decades and that continued growth is unwarranted. Some economists agree that health care spending has contributed to the overall increase in the GNP. Paul Starr has written, "Since 1970 the economic stakes in the battle over health care have risen sharply. In 1970 *Business Week* called health care a '$60 billion crisis'; by 1991 the cost was approaching—and now exceeds—$800 billion a year. Health care spending had risen from 7.3% to 13.2% of GNP. Since 1980, health care has consumed an additional 1% of GNP every 35 months."[2] Since then, the government has examined and continues to seek reforms for health care funding and management. The presentation of these reform proposals has spawned more private marketplace solutions, in the form of IDSs, to both increase quality and keep costs low. Although an integrated health care organization can provide seamless health care delivery systems, it is tricky to develop an organization that can handle the acquisition and management of new and unfamiliar businesses. In addition, integrated health care organizations need to demonstrate compelling benefits for the marketplace.

Health care delivery has evolved, shaped by the funding directions of government payers, private payers, and managed care payers. As providers take increasing risks in payment and service delivery, the economic and operational purposes for the formation of integrated organizations becomes more relevant. The rules and shapes of allocation of resources—from government, private payers, and managed care payers—have also changed. Historically, health care providers have sought resources from these areas and have shaped themselves to maximize reimbursement. From the earliest policies that funded health care delivery to more recent decades that encouraged the move to free market enterprise, the delivery system has been shaped by resource requirements.

PLANNING AS A TOOL FOR BEING PREPARED

In the wake of these changes, the best way to proceed is to be prepared. To be effective, the planning process involves obtaining strategic information, forming a vision, and anticipating opportunities. A meaningful planning process provides a design to chart directions, improve services, and maximize reimbursement according to available resources. Theodore Levitt described why organizations plan: "Regarding the future, where, indeed, we will have to spend the rest of our lives, the necessity for action cannot be avoided by flight into rhetoric or isolation into analysis. We must get organized for action. Study, calculation, and budgeting reduce uncertainty and transform it into risk. We may have to study and calculate faster, but also with more reliance on the common sense that nature, wisdom and experience confer. Experience comes from what we have done, wisdom from what we have done badly."[3]

There are for-profit management firms for hospitals and physician practices. Characteristically, these firms are diversified among many markets, although some are concentrated in specific regions of the country. With many concurrent negotiations in place to enter a market, one of the hallmarks of the successful for-profit firms is their ability to enter more quickly into arrangements than the less well-positioned organizations. The strategic position is the prepared position, and planning is an essential strategic tool for reaching this position. Stan Davis, a leading business thinker, wrote about the challenges that lie ahead: "As business migrates toward the economic value of knowledge, as both provider and consumer, its organizations will move in the same direction. The characteristics of these organizations, therefore, seem certain: a focus on service and productivity, increasingly fast, flexible, customized networked and global."[4]

For the organization to be successful, it must be prepared to

- move with opportunities for success
- work with multiple contingencies
- achieve organizational self-knowledge and assessment
- move fast and intelligently
- know the key players in the marketplace

In short, it must plan for the development of organizational relationships and relationship management. Development of these skills and knowledge will allow access to markets and community groups when trying to extend access to services without having to duplicate market channels.

Move with Opportunities for Success

The importance of planning for the future is, and has been, to be prepared to move with opportunities for success. Success is driven by being prepared to pursue, avail oneself of, and respond to opportunities. Management expert Theodore Levitt has said, "It is not so much the accurately forecasted future we need as attentiveness and quick response to the forces that are shaping today's events and environment."[5] One industry analyst has seen in Columbia/HCA's rapid style of acquisition the strategy of preparedness:

- a well-prepared, very experienced acquisition team
- an aggressive and persistent approach
- unusual speed and flexibility in deal-making
- a reputation for not overvaluing acquisitions[6]

Columbia/HCA has been extremely successful in entering a market, becoming a significant player in it by acquiring a critical mass of care facilities (hospital and ambulatory surgery centers), and then building regional delivery systems to support those acquisitions. This consistent goal, with a customized approach for each region, equals strategic preparedness. Other progressive firms, including Tenet Healthcare and Phy-Cor, also are known for using this strategy.

Work with Multiple Contingencies

Planning provides the road map for an organization to meet the anticipated clinical practice challenges, develop marketplaces, and gain new customer groups to improve market position. Planning also provides a process and mechanism to unite the range of professionals involved in a health care delivery system to move in a strategic direction. Increasingly, complex organizations located in complex markets find that their strategies include multiple contingencies. For example, Meridia Health System, Cleveland, Ohio, negotiated with several potential partners simultaneously prior to their merger with the Cleveland Clinic. The strategic plan of New England Medical Center (NEMC), Boston, Massachusetts, identified several potential partners with whom they had concurrent explorations. LifeSpan, with whom they eventually merged, was not a first-round candidate for merger. However, when it later emerged as an affiliation option, NEMC's preparedness allowed it to come together in a matter of weeks.

Achieve Organizational Self-Knowledge and Assessment

The health care organization, historically focused on one or more hospitals and increasingly including employed—rather than affiliated—physicians, is traditionally encumbered by costs and demands that prevent rapid response to community needs and market opportunities. Therefore, planning in a chaotic environment, with vision, innovation, and rapid response, requires organizational self-knowledge and assessment. A strategy development and update process can be useful.

The more preparation done for strategic planning (in assessing both the internal and external environments), the more flexible is the organization's ability to adapt to changes in those environments. One needs to know the organization's strengths and weaknesses—in facilities, personnel, and services offered. The more self-knowledge the organization has, the faster that organization can respond to new challenges and opportunities. In a changing environment such as health care delivery, rapid responses to challenges and flexible adaptation to change are key factors for success.

Move Fast and Intelligently

The ability to assess the internal organization is critical. Organizational self-knowledge calls for a theoretical and practical understanding of the current position and options in a strategic and tactical sense. It is about being ready to move fast and intelligently. Knowing an organization well creates the opportunity to respond to challenges. Requiring time for research before formulating an action plan can allow opportunities to slip by.

Many organizations have used the self-assessment or internal assessment to determine the efficiency of their delivery of health care services. Chapter 3 of this book further explores the environmental assessment.

Know the Key Players in the Marketplace

Being prepared includes having an understanding of the players (people and organizations) in the marketplace—their services, their capabilities, and their needs. That includes constituencies with which the hospital has regular contact—physicians, employees, insurers, employers, and primary customers. It also includes those that often act on the periphery of the hospital environment—social service agencies, local health departments, schools, and other agencies.

INTEGRATING THE ORGANIZATION'S STRATEGIC DIRECTIONS INTO A STRATEGIC PLAN

Strategic directions help the management team to navigate the organization through a course designed to achieve its strategic vision. The integration of strategic directions with the management agenda raises the likelihood that intended outcomes will be achieved. The useful strategic plan is neither a document on the shelf nor a list of goals and objectives. The strategic plan shows the team where the organization wants to go, how to get there, what price the organization is willing to pay, and what concessions it is or is not willing to make. The implementation of the plan as a management process, and the later evaluation of the planning activity, help guide the organization while yielding desired results. The strategic plan articulates the organization's direction through the vision statement and the stated intended actions. Strategy, based on a methodological, practical review of information, also directs an organization toward a vision of what it can become. See chapter 2 for a more thorough exploration of the strategic plan.

Because the plan without action is useless, organizational leadership, as the means of guiding the workforce to attain innovations throughout the organization, has never been more important. Plan development engages the leadership, provides an opportunity to review previous trends, learn from other providers, and create a vision for the organization's future. When the plan has been developed and approved, the implementation stage includes articulation of the strategies, providing for the functional ability to execute the new directions, and enabling the activation of the intended accomplishments.

Strategies Designed to Meet Unique Marketplace Demands

Each marketplace demands a unique strategy. For example, the supply of health care providers and primary care physicians may indicate the influx of more physicians. The presence of managed care firms may indicate provider readiness to operate under capitation. *The Dartmouth Atlas of Health Care* reviewed 306 health care markets around the country and assessed the differences in costs and health care use in each. The variability in these markets reflects the variety in arrangements between providers and payers. Employers are using such data sets because of their interest in the variation in the cost of health care across the country. Mary Jane England, M.D., president of the Washington Business Group on Health, has expressed concern with the drive toward standardization: "Although we support standardizing information for purchasers, employers must use that information in the context of the community, which has its own demographics and culture."[7]

A corporate customer may be paying various rates for the same services in different markets. Medicare payments from the Health Care Financing Administration (HCFA) also respond to individual markets. The capitation rates, paid on the basis of area-adjusted per-capita cost (AAPCC) rates, respond to individual markets. Employers are behind the development and use of the Health Plan Employer Data and Information Set (HEDIS) data set from National Committee for Quality Assurance

(NCQA). The data set was developed for commercially insured populations, while variations due to Medicare and Medicaid enrollees are incorporated in version 3.0 of HEDIS. The latest versions will facilitate plan-to-plan comparison, although the longitudinal comparison will be complicated. Nonetheless, the variety of markets and the variety of circumstances in each market require tailored answers and deliberate strategy to maximize health care delivery and payment, and to ensure garnering market share that will support the health care organization. Management expert Peter Drucker has commented, "Corporate size will by the end of the coming decade have become a strategic decision. Neither 'big is better' nor 'small is beautiful' makes much sense. . . . Size follows function. . . . Management will increasingly have to decide on the right size for a business, the size that fits its technology, its strategy and its markets."[8]

There are several versions of stages of consolidation, stages of managed care development, and stages of levels of competitiveness. Health care provider strategy and payer strategy both hinge on market characteristics and recommended tactics for effective competition. Strategy is both attending to the characteristics of the local marketplace and having a comprehensive view of the organization—the better to assess opportunities and directions.

The approach to acquisition in each market depends on each marketplace. National provider organizations that operate in many markets, such as PhyCor, Physicians Quality Care, Tenet Healthcare, and Columbia/HCA, tailor their approaches to the characteristics of the marketplace. In that way, the for-profit firm, which has a uniform goal and a variety of means of achieving objectives, will shape its approach and entry into a marketplace according to the regional players' perceptions and interests.

Insights Provided by National Trend Reports

Environmental updates and trend reports profile recent and emerging activities in the health care provider industries. All of these provide some level of insight into what is happening at a macro level in the industry. Providers must recognize trends. They must understand how trends in other markets affect the local market, and how local participants are likely to react. Leveraging knowledge of national trends can allow a health care organization to lead through innovation and to compete through the strategic management of information.

Variation in Managed Care Penetration Annual updates on managed care activity show that managed care penetration ranges from 0 percent to more than 40 percent of the HMO population. Other studies show that because customers have a greater choice of providers, enrollment in PPOs is growing at a faster rate than that of HMOs. Other findings note that in some large metropolitan areas, managed care activity is significantly different than the statewide volumes quoted.

National payers and national research firms have noted variation in the degree of penetration of the for-profit health care management firms in different markets. Markets differ; role-model areas may have more or less managed care, more or less integration, and more or less integration of health care providers. In short, "if you have seen one market, you have seen only one market." Any planning must take these variations into account.

Changes in Health Care Network Structures Although health care reform has been on many political and business agendas in the past several years, it is clear that the health care industry needs to plan for multiple levels of change and for some level of selection of services. The *New York Times* noted that despite the Clinton Administration's legislative failure to transform American medicine, the actual proposal may have served as a catalyst for change:

> HMOs are booming: more than 58 million Americans are enrolled in prepaid health plans. Three in four doctors have converted at least part of their private practice into work for the HMOs and health care companies that increasingly control the supply of patients and the cost of treatments. Patrician medical establishments—like Massachusetts General Hospital in Boston and New York Hospital–Cornell Medical Center in Manhattan—that once seemed impervious to commercial pressures are racing into mergers to guarantee their survival. In some respects, it is what the Clintons' army of health care cognoscenti envisioned: medicine made more affordable by a long-overdue dose of competition.[9]

Participants in the formation of the Clinton proposal agree that the anticipation of government-enacted capitation became a catalyst for organizations to prepare for nationwide capitation. Changes include the emergence of organizational structures best suited for capitation—IDSs.[10]

Changes in the structure of health care networks affect physicians and hospitals more than they do the payers and suppliers. Many providers cite their need to integrate in order to attract managed care contracts. At the same time, the increased presence of managed care and the transition of Medicare and Medicaid enrollees into HMOs is yet another way for government to facilitate a more competitive market.

Changes in Provider Relationships The relationships have shifted between and among providers and between providers and payers over the last several decades. Most important, there is a greater level of consolidation. Several factors brought about this change. Since the 1980s, the health care delivery system has emphasized hospital-physician bonding. In the past decade, as each entity has moved into the business of employing physicians and managing practices, the financial stability of primary care providers has become more of a focal point for both hospitals and payers attempting to gain and keep market share. Integration has increased. The payers' stronger relationships with selected acute care providers create incentives for providers to drive costs down through integration.

Shift in Economic Incentives for Providers   The popularity of capitation as a potential means of decreasing costs for employers has enabled Medicare and Medicaid to change from managing acute care to managing lives. This change signaled a profound shift in economic incentives for health care providers, moving from counting disease encounters (hospitalizations, lengths of stay, physician visit encounters), to counting enrollees in a plan assigned to a particular primary care provider (counting health status measures and management protocols).

Capitation also represents a change from viewing the hospital as a revenue center to a cost center. Instead of a hospital providing the bulk of health care services, its use is minimized for cost management purposes. Services preceding and following acute care have grown and will continue to grow as a means of decreasing health care expenses. The incorporation of alternative medicine also will continue to grow as an alternative to traditional medical care. With these changes in health care delivery during this period and the subsequent paradigm shift, physicians and acute care providers and payers have moved into each others' spheres of business. They have done so in order to provide the maximum amount of flexibility in attracting and keeping business. The anticipated increase of capitation in many markets and the need to manage decreasing payments more creatively have prompted integration as a means of long-term economic stability.

The Strategic Plan and the Organization's Vision and Values

The founding mission states the organization's purpose for being. The vision tells when the company intends to position itself in the marketplace, and what community it intends to serve and on what level. The strategic plan directs the life of the organization. It outlines how it will reach that future while staying true to its founding mission. For each step of the plan, one needs to ask, Will this move us toward our vision? Is this part of the mission? The vision is more loosely written than a definite description of the organization, and it serves to guide the organization in negotiating and positioning in its environment. Theodore Levitt has neatly summarized the importance of vision. "The world is run mostly by emotion and justified by calculation," he writes. "The future of your enterprise depends largely on the interplay between invention and vision, between technological capability and entrepreneurial quest, between the social dream and the organizational system in which the dream resides."[11]

The mix of vision, mission, values, and strategy is an interactive one. The organization's values dictate the "how" of its strategy—how the vision will be accomplished, how people will work with one another, and how the goals will be attained. Commitment to the community is traditionally a part of the values (as reflected in the mission), and the organization's services ideally respond to community need. The values also affect the health care delivery system's policy and financing.

The use of vision, mission, and values statements as guides for organizational direction and priority are new to health care delivery, but they are not new to successful business organizations. As tools, they are an integral part of inculcating and aligning employees' and affiliated physicians' attitudes and goals with the future of the organization.

The Strategic Plan and Organizational Commitment to the Community   Commitment to the mission statement usually has roots in commitment to the community. Recent emphasis on public health indicators suggests a comprehensive approach to statistical data and collaboration. Healthy community issues may address physical health, real or perceived access to health care, quality of life, safety, and environmental conditions and programs that ultimately improve the local economy.

These changes in health care arise from pressure on society and the economy, and they reflect changes in society's perspectives on itself— namely, a spirit of community commitment. This commitment to solving societal problems means coming together as a community, within a community, and appropriately responding to the needs of the community. This ethos is also incorporated by employer groups or coalitions and not just by geographically defined community groups.

Capitation payment shifts clinical management and payment to providers, requiring demonstrated value of managing the health care needs not only of the enrollees but of the defined community. The responsibility for the community is part of most not-for-profit health care organizations' mission statements, developed in the articles of incorporation, and maintained in the securement of the not-for-profit status. Behind the inherent independence of clinical care management under capitation, which grants great independence in providing clinical care, one of the safeguards in protecting the community is to monitor the health of the community.

Community health care underpinned the Clinton health reform proposal. According to Nancy Dubler, cochair of The Ethical Foundation of the New System Working Group, the committee based their recommendations on the concept of *communitarianism*—under which the problems faced by members of a community are responded to by other members.[12] For example, underserved groups in urban areas (such as unregistered immigrants) and residents in rural areas face differing access challenges and require different solutions.

If health care is viewed as a social good at a statewide level, then care for the uninsured is shared by providers and payers. Competitive pricing is inhibited when some organizations are committed to funding free care and others are not. One solution may be to arrive at a policy to determine who pays into a central fund that provides care for those who cannot afford it. A different solution may be chosen, locally or by the health care industry as a whole.

PLANNING'S ROLE IN THE DEVELOPMENT OF HEALTH CARE SERVICE DELIVERY

The health care industry has been driven by

- government policies that funded health care delivery
- the insurance industry that provided rapid payment through employer channels and premiums
- the public reaction to health care access
- the emergence of prepaid health care

Hospitals and physicians face national forces that encourage their coming together, either with each other or with other entities. The benefits of collaboration are decreased costs and enhanced services to customer groups.

Planning has gone beyond building facilities and now includes providing locally controlled care, developing competitive strategy, preparing for regional capitation, creating IDSs, and developing value-driven market-oriented organizations. The structure of federal funding drove the development of medical education, acute care facilities, and community health centers, while coordinated community planning required proof of the use of the resources. The decrease in federal or state resources drove the onset of competition in health care organizations, which fostered cost decreases, emphasis on core competencies, and greater focus on efficient alignments. The shift in health care delivery consideration toward greater responsibility for the community has resulted in societal solutions outside acute medical care and a demonstrated commitment to the health of communities—health maintenance. Payers' current demand for low cost and choice of providers has directed planning to a competitive and often collaborative position.

Heavy regulation in the health care delivery system over the past several years has resulted in planning in health care that focused on resource attainment and revenue maximization in a regulated environment. As the government payers and private payers shift their incentives, seeking to decrease health care costs and increase overall service value, further changes in health care delivery trends will result.

Government programs have historically funded health care delivery services. Through government policy and programs, health care services built facilities, purchased equipment, built medical schools, and paid for new services. Historically, the planning function has been charged with getting those new resources. As changing government policies have moved from payment of capital to increasing market competition, the planning function has similarly evolved to maximize service delivery and stabilize revenue.

Planning in the 1940s and 1950s: Build It and They Will Come

The Great Depression brought massive unemployment, resulting in federal policies creating jobs. During World War II, more than 11 million Americans served in the military, using government-provided facilities, which created a sense of government services. Coupled with the GI bill and housing assistance, a new image of government emerged in public expectations. The postwar era was a time of demand for material products to support the American dream—where everyone was to have a car and a house. This era brought about significant changes in the social and economic landscape. For example, changes in federal taxation rewarded home ownership and created incentives for moving out of urban rental properties. Suburban housing areas sprang up, attracting young homeowners and creating bedroom communities where people lived who commuted to urban jobs. Within these suburbs, demand increased for localized health care and other services. Government policies created incentives for such local health care delivery.

Thus, the health care industry grew as a reflection of government policy and economic direction. According to a 1943 poll, people thought it was a "good idea" for Social Security to pay for doctor and hospital care.[13] With increased mass communication, health care issues came into a greater public focus. The polio epidemic of the 1950s held public attention as the battle against polio became a public cause. While television and radio spread information about its impact on children, they also alerted the public about long lines for vaccinations. Ultimately, this experience changed the public expectations of health care. People wanted solutions in their towns, schools, and medical institutions. Investment in local public health programs meant that government would pay for it—directly or indirectly. Although there was increased pressure for entitled services in 1950, health care costs were only approximately 4.6 percent of the gross national product.[14]

The Payers In the midst of postwar growth was discussion of national health insurance (although it was recommended for study rather than legislative action). By 1946, President Truman signed into law the Hospital Survey and Construction Act. Although health care reform ultimately was not enacted, government payments were allowed for hospital construction and research funds for medical schools. In fact, investments in medical schools were enormous in the 1940s; the average income for a medical school grew from $500,000 per year in the 1940s to $3.7 million in the late 1950s. The medical schools became large, complex organizations with a mission focused on research, education, and patient care.[15] With growth came differentiation and specialization.

Hospital planning called for facility expansion and services based on the scientific and technological interest of clinicians. Planning was typically conducted by facility managers, who handled construction, and clinicians, who planned their next renovation or addition. Greater availability of hospital resources shifted the inpatient population dramatically from the critically ill to the moderately ill, from the difficult maternity case to the general maternity case. The perspective of the consumer was that making services available would inevitably build up the demand. Roemer and Shain's 1959 study concluded that the increase of hospital beds raised the use of hospitals by the insured population. The planning of services focused on facility development.

During this period, private insurance companies started to grow. By 1939, hospital payment plans were governed by state-specific legislation. The majority of the directors represented hospitals and allowed the insurance commissioners rate review authority in exchange for being designated tax-exempt. Blue Cross organizations had the privileged tax exemptions and relationships with hospitals, creating a market advantage over commercial insurance companies. By 1940, insurance companies had nearly 4 million subscribers, while the 39 Blue Cross plans had a total enrollment of more than 6 million.[16] Commercial insurers started experience rating, which allowed them to have lower rates, and the rest of the insurance industry followed the practice. This left the aged and poor to the government payment system. Private insurance offered a different kind of financial security than did government programs and a speedier cash flow to physicians and hospitals.

The Buyers By the early 1940s, several prepayment plans or health care cooperatives had started up—with the majority represented by physicians. The growth of organized labor made a difference in how employers paid for health care, by expanding the scope of coverage and reducing employee contributions. As of 1945, on average, employers paid 10 percent of the cost of insurance; by 1950, collective bargaining agreements required them to pay 37 percent of the employee cost and 20 percent for dependents.[17] During this time, the unions changed the nature of insurance. Paul Starr, in *The Social Transformation of American Medicine,* has written, "The union shop, which in the early fifties made union membership mandatory for more than two thirds of the production work force, enabled the unions to establish a 'private fiscal system' able to levy a 'tax' for health insurance."[18]

Unions were a major force in developing prepaid group practices to ensure benefits for members and their families. In the 1940s, union negotiations also had a role in the development of prepaid managed care, with Community Health Centers of Two Harbors, Minnesota; Labor Health Institute of St. Louis; and Miners' Clinics in Pennsylvania, Ohio, and West Virginia. Outside organized labor, health insurance became a fringe benefit of employment. In addition, the growth in real incomes in these two decades allowed more access to medical services.

The Providers This period brought development of prepaid group practices. Kaiser Health Plan, started in the early 1940s, was established to provide prepaid medical care for shipyard workers and their families—with one plan in Portland, Oregon, and the other in Oakland, California. At the end of World War II, these programs were nearly closed, but opening enrollment to other employers in 1945 ensured Kaiser's success.

This period also saw increased funding for hospitals. After 1945, as policy makers looked toward the future of the economy in the postwar period, the direction of science and medicine increased jobs (in construction and new technology) and local medical services. The federal government facilitated the distribution of health resources, with the 1946 Hill-Burton program (the Hospital Survey and Construction Act) expanding rural hospitals. A federally mandated program, Hill-Burton was administered by the states, who, it was believed, would be better able to manage the resource allocation according to regional needs. The act did not encourage coordination among the hospitals or increase their economic stability.

Between 1947 and 1971, Hill-Burton disbursed $3.7 billion for construction and generated approximately $9.1 billion from other sources. As of 1971, more than 75 percent of those moneys went to hospitals. In 1954 a modification to the program added long-term care and ambulatory facilities to other facilities.

Through the late 1950s, hospitals sought affiliations with medical schools to attract interns and residents. Subsequently, the medical schools increased their influence in the hospital systems of metropolitan areas. Notably, the price of hospital care doubled during the 1950s. The greater need for the hospitals by those more than 65 years old contributed to the groundswell of interest for a health insurance program for those on Social Security. The postwar era was a time of greater public expectation that the federal government would provide medical services. The health care industry grew, as did health care costs.

Planning in the 1960s and 1970s: A Focus on the Community

In the 1960s, national leadership brought the idealism of social responsibility to both international and domestic initiatives. The start of the Peace Corps as well as the domestic war on poverty, created a decade filled with programs focused on community-based action—whether that community was a city, state, country, or continent. This belief that America could solve problems around the world fostered confidence that led to building a Great Society, with a war on poverty planned during the Kennedy administration and implemented in the Johnson administration.

The Great Society programs of the early and mid-1960s shifted the health care landscape to include new payers and new providers, Medicare and Medicaid. The newly funded providers, Community Health Centers, were located in underserved rural and urban areas. The acute care providers were also responsible for education and other services based on consumer need. In response to the greater demand for health services and new advances in medicine, a 1959 government report expressed concern about an impending physician shortage, noting that medical schools would need to increase from 7,400 graduates per year to 11,000 graduates per year to preserve physician-to-population ratios. There also was a nursing shortage, and in 1963 the first series of measures to aid and expand health professional education was adopted.

Awareness of rising medical costs started to surface during the late 1960s. Based on the 52 percent cost increases in 20 years, from 4.6 percent of the GNP in 1950 to 7 percent of the GNP in 1970, voices from both the government and the press declared a crisis in the escalation of health care costs:

- In July 1969, President Nixon, speaking about the rapidly escalating costs in Medicare and Medicaid, announced, "We face a massive crisis in this area. Unless action is taken . . . we will have a breakdown in our medical system."
- In January 1970, *Business Week* ran a cover story on the $60 billion crisis and compared medical care in America unfavorably with national health programs elsewhere in the western world.
- In January 1970, *Fortune* declared that American medicine stood "on the brink of chaos."[19]

Following are the most important health care measures adopted in this period:

- *Graduate Medical Education National Advisory Committee (GMENAC):* In 1976, the Department of Health Education and Welfare created the GMENAC, which projected for 1990 the need for physicians, by specialty, using demographic, epidemiological, scientific, and technological trend data. The results showed an anticipated surplus of physicians, with shortages predicted in a few areas (psychiatry, emergency medicine, and preventive medicine), as well as an inefficient geographic distribution of physicians. Competition became clear with the identification of a physician surplus in some areas.[20]

- *Medicare and Medicaid:* Despite extensive earlier efforts to introduce some version of an insurance plan for people more than 65 years of age, Medicare wasn't approved until 1964, even though it was a priority in the Great Society programs. Part A provided compulsory hospital insurance, while Part B provided government-subsidized voluntary insurance for physician care. The third component was Medicaid, which expanded assistance to the states for medical care for the poor, all signed into law on July 30, 1965. While initiated together, the Medicare and Medicaid programs differed. Medicare, supported by popular approval and tied to Society Security participation, was federally overseen and allowed physicians to charge more than the stated reimbursement levels. In contrast, Medicaid had the stigma of public assistance, was overseen by the states, and required providers to pay established fee levels.

- *1966 Community Planning Legislation:* The 1966 Community Planning Legislation started Community Health Centers, creating full-service primary care centers in low-income areas. The Centers employed local residents and had community participation in overseeing the Centers. The objective was to develop indigenous capabilities and leadership and was part of the War on Poverty's focus on capabilities development. Sponsorship and support came from medical schools, local hospitals, and health departments. By 1967, community health centers were viewed as the major providers for the poor. With the expansion of the Medicaid budget, the growth of the centers was halted. At the same time, Hill-Burton and the community mental health center program was refocused to support health care in low-income areas.

- *Comprehensive Health Planning and Public Health Service Amendments Act of 1966* and the *National Health Planning and Resources Development Act of 1974:* State and regional planning started with passage of the Comprehensive Health Planning and Public Health Service Amendments Act of 1966, and the National Health Planning and Resources Development Act of 1974. These resulted in significant changes, such as the formation of the national and regional planning agencies, State Health Planning and Development Agencies (SHPDAs) and regional Health System Areas

(HSAs). These agencies established criteria for and then reviewed and approved capital investments, in the form of renovation, equipment, and new services through regulations pertaining to certificates and determination of need. Many hospitals, faced with new regulatory complexities, staffed their organizations with planners, familiar with both regulatory compliance requirements and program planning techniques.

- *Federal utilization review program:* In the 1970s, cost-savings measures were started with the federal government's utilization review program as a check on physician and hospital treatment and billing. Because it was conducted retrospectively, it did not influence the delivery of care or help with quality assurance; it only limited reimbursement. The health care planning agencies, who reviewed and approved capital investment decisions of the hospitals, did not direct resources prior to their use.

Also, during this period, the continual growth of insurance as a benefit of employment contributed to increased access to medical care. Major payers—Medicare, Medicaid, and Blue Cross—paid hospitals based on their costs. Since Medicare paid physicians based on "customary" fees, it created incentives to increase charges and physician fees climbed. Prevailing charges in geographic areas rewarded physicians located in high-priced areas.

The Providers   Because of the capital investment provided by the Hill-Burton program, the enforced coordination from the regulatory process, and Medicare's reimbursement of depreciation, hospital growth was assured. The depreciation reimbursement guaranteed the continuation of services and also meant that the largest and newest hospitals received the most depreciation reimbursement.

Although most health care delivery organizations were organized as not-for-profits, the seed for development of for-profit health care delivery started in 1969, when Hospital Corporation of America went public and was successful in its offering. With that, the concept of well-managed hospitals operating on a for-profit basis was off to an infamous start. The rise of hospital membership organizations is further evidence of provider integration and affiliation. The organizations provided purchasing cooperatives and forums to share information and expertise. For example, the Voluntary Hospitals of America alliance started with 30 not-for-profit facilities in 1977.

Practice gave way to the profession of planning, as evidenced by the start in 1978 of the American Hospital Association personal membership group known as the Society for Hospital Planning. Planning was focused on regulatory compliance, applications for new technology, community needs assessment, and the best use of statistical indicators and demographic data. Its focus expanded to include subjective information from community advisory groups.

As far as prepaid group practices were concerned, HMOs were recognized as a possible means of controlling the rapid increase in cost and utilization of health care services. The 1967 document, *A Report to the President on Medical Care Prices,* identified HMOs as a possible means of controlling costs.[21] By 1970, the Nixon Administration became interested in prepaid health care and, in 1971, the first HMO bill was introduced. The Health Maintenance Organization Act of 1973 authorized development assistance to HMOs, anticipating eventual self-sufficiency. The law provided financial aid for development and growth and provided funds for expansion into medically underserved areas. HMO access was supported by contracts for retired military and federal employees. The Society Security Amendment of 1972 strengthened the relationship between Medicare and HMOs by establishing Medicare programs on a cost reimbursement basis and by allowing for HMO contracts with Medicaid.

Health care services grew under the coordination of the state planning agencies through the certificate-of-need process. With cost-based reimbursement by both government and insurance payers, there were few incentives to create real value for the purchasers of health care services. The hospitals had economic and medical service incentives to acquire technology—creating what has been called a "medical arms race" for technology and service capability. While the medical industry grew, the subsequent cost increases became the target of federal and state governments, as well as the public. The search for alternatives led to the introduction of managed care. From the consumer perspective, the indemnity insurance was a security blanket to use for growing local health care resources.

Planning in the 1980s: The Customer Is Always Right

The tone of the 1980s was one of affluence and easy access to money. The new federal administration starting the decade was one in which there were reductions of government's role in service delivery and a great reliance on market competition and appropriate incentives. Planning during this period became focused on survival strategies for health care organizations. Institutions responded to declining use rates of hospital inpatient services with initiatives toward market share gain, program development, and quality integration. Relatively little formal collaboration or merger activity took place at this time.

If concerns over the health care costs were high in 1970, they were even higher in the 1980s. From 1970 to 1980, health care expenses grew from 7.2 percent of the GNP to 9.4 percent—a 31 percent jump. In actual numbers, the industry went from $69 billion to $230 billion in those 10 years.[22]

The Payers The greater interest level in HMOs as a mode of shifting risk to the private sector was demonstrated when HMO oversight was moved from the Public Health Service to the HCFA Office of Prepaid Healthcare in 1982. Congressional passage of the Tax Equity and Fiscal Responsibility Act of 1982 initiated HCFA's payments to HMOs on a capitated basis for Medicare enrollees. In 1983, reimbursement to hospitals for Medicare enrollees changed from fee-for-service to fixed rates through diagnosis-related groups (DRGs), providing the incentives to hospitals to offset inpatient care with outpatient care.

In the 1980s, insurance took hold as a major perk for employees. At the same time, payers such as HCFA changed from fee-for-service payments to hospitals to fixed-rate reimbursement, regardless of cost or length of stay. Other payers followed and moved to case-rate reimbursement or even per diem payments. Inpatient care was carefully supplemented by outpatient care for which there were no such payment constraints, and hospitals started moving into the outpatient acute care business as well as the inpatient acute care business.

The Providers The predicted growth of corporate medicine brought about the rise of large health care corporations. A 1980 editorial in the *New England Journal of Medicine* noted "the rise of a new medical-industrial complex."[23] The lessons learned from private corporate businesses used in nonprofit health care led to five changes:

- *type of ownership and control:* the shift from nonprofit and governmental organizations to for-profit companies in health care
- *horizontal integration:* the rise of multi-institutional systems and a consequent shift to the locus of control from community boards to regional and national health care corporations
- *diversification and corporate restructuring:* the shift from single-unit organizations operating in one market to "polycorporate," sometimes with both nonprofit and for-profit subsidiaries involved in a variety of different health care markets
- *vertical integration:* the shift from single-level-of-care organizations, such as acute care hospitals, to organizations that embrace the various phases and levels of care, such as HMOs
- *industry concentration:* the increasing concentration of ownership and control of health services in regional markets and the nation as a whole

These trends represent the increased merger activity from which price controls and service enhancements were expected. However, with a deregulated environment, the push for horizontal integration soon moved to a surge of activities supporting vertical integration. In search of proven economic superiority, health care organizations amalgamated, shifted care to the ambulatory setting, and converted inpatient resources to a full spectrum of pre- and post–acute care services.

In the 1980s, the industry trend was to develop a full range of services for "cradle-to-grave" capabilities. With the growth of diversification came greater emphasis on new business development. The business development of the full spectrum of services was part of the search for both greater market share and market dominance as part of a deregulated environment.

Health care continued to diversify into related and unrelated businesses. Hospitals merged and formed holding companies to be able to develop other corporations under one umbrella, giving rise to the start of "health care systems." In 1981, three for-profit hospital management companies dominated the for-profit multihospital systems: HCA, Humana, and American Medical International.

The move to enhance quality services was part of the change in health care delivery. Rapid change in competitive pressures, shifts in the setting of care delivery, and a renewed focus on the consumer required careful oversight of quality. Quality of service delivery became a new focus, and managers sought to apply total quality management and continual quality improvement initiatives to health care.[24]

The challenge to planning was to be more responsive to the market by developing competitive strategies to obtain market share (and increase volume), as the best means of growth and support for the hospital. Accordingly, understanding the consumer expectations of provider selection became essential to formulating a competitive strategy. Other important steps were using forecasting services, product development, and using regulatory support for capital acquisition. Heightened attention went to relating more closely with physicians (physician bonding programs), payers (managed care contracting strategies), and purchasers (direct contracting).

The emphasis on market forces refocused attention on community-based planning. This emphasis recalled the values from the 1960s to make health care available. The drive for market share by hospitals was seen as a universal solution to the declining inpatient census and admissions. The shift in professional practice was reflected in an organizational change: The American Society for Hospital Public Relations—later the American Society for Healthcare Marketing and Public Relations— merged with the Society for Healthcare Planning and Marketing in 1996, to become the Society for Healthcare Strategy and Market Development.

Prepaid health care delivery also evolved in this period. It was thought that the growth of managed care as an employee benefit would decrease health care costs. The market opportunity of increased volume through managed care contracts led to greater involvement of the providers in prepaid health care delivery systems. The staff model plans experienced declining growth compared to PPOs and independent practice associations. Clearly, provider choice was important in the marketplace. In addition, regional market penetration by managed care plans grew; the regions and states with higher penetration were examined by providers in other parts of the country to see how they fared, both financially and clinically.

Planning in the 1990s: Planning for Market Conditions

The business perspective on health care shifted from diversification because that strategy yielded poor financial returns. The new focus was core competencies, with an increased emphasis on demonstrated quality and capabilities. The failure of speculative financial markets led to a refocus on personal values and new attitudes toward disposable income, as well as renewed emphasis on family, as the baby boom generation raised its own children.

Hospitals and health networks have responded to market forces by establishing cost-containment measures and procedures that correspond to capitation requirements. Management examines and reconfigures clinical delivery systems to achieve the expected cost position. Further, the pressure to secure a primary care network (including covered lives or affiliated customers) has spawned physician practice acquisition by providers, payers, and suppliers. Many of the practices operate at significant losses, though the losses are offset by other revenue streams.

Per capita spending for health care rose significantly in the last decade and is projected to grow in spite of slower growth in other sectors of the economy. Most of these increases resulted from inflation instead of volume increases or service quality improvements, according to HCFA.

The Payers The desire to stem health care inflation, running at nearly 12 percent annually, facilitated interest in health reform. The health care industry could either allow market forces to handle the inflation challenges or let the government set global payment rates and establish rates and standards. While many experts pushed hard for government controls, such legislation was defeated because of the cost to the system and the limitation of choice.

In the early part of the decade, the industry prepared for capitation, or at least a capitation system regulated by a national health insurance plan. The Clinton Administration health care reform proposal suggested a model of managed competition with a national health board, and state and regional health alliances (or corporate alliances) that would contract with health care providers. Accountable health plans would form to organize hospitals, doctors, and other health service providers into regional or corporate alliances. Preparations for a massive level of capitation encouraged providers to work together to form more coordinated services and focused attention on consolidation. Following this preparation, states took greater initiative, and health care delivery organizations started to form integrated systems to attract capitated contracts.

During this period, managed care plans grew and merged to gain greater market advantage. In 1990, Cigna acquired Equicor, a joint venture of the Equitable Life Assurance Society and HCA. Travelers and Metropolitan's managed care business merged to become MetraHealth Company, which was then acquired by United HealthCare Corp. Aetna acquired US Healthcare to move into the managed care business rapidly. Kaiser Permanente started to implement plans to affiliate with Group Health Cooperative of Puget Sound. Payers wanting to improve their own distribution channels started investing in physician networks in the early 1990s. Those firms included Cigna, Prudential, Aetna Health Plans, MetLife Healthcare, and United Healthcare. The insurers moving into managed care enter the market either by developing plans from their indemnity capabilities or by acquiring prepaid plans.

Finally, reports of the increasing number of people participating in managed care plans are met with a variety of reactions. From the employers who receive an economic advantage, there may be a search for demonstrated value and relief from the decreased costs. In 1995, a Foster Higgins study reported that an HMO enrollee paid approximately $804 less than an enrollee in a traditional indemnity insurance program, bringing home the point that it is cheaper to have employees participate in managed care. By early 1996, 58.2 million persons were enrolled in approximately 600 HMOs.[25]

The Providers   From fee-for-service, to case rates under DRGs, to global capitation, the emphasis shifts depending on the strategy of the moment. Disease management has become important, with the increasing attention of case managers looking at guideline-based treatment, outcomes management, and total quality improvement. Planners are directing the coordination of care across all spectrums of care as health care delivery organizations move toward capitation and medical management.

In 1995, National Medical Enterprise merged with AMI to become Tenet Healthcare, which has since merged with OrNda, becoming the second-largest for-profit hospital management company. Even as merger explorations take place with Columbia/HCA, the consolidation trend continues. The opportunity to consolidate providers in the same organized fashion that national payer and managed care organizations enjoy exists for the new structures of providers. The stand-alone physician practices and hospitals that are not organized (characteristic of a cottage industry) are being urged to participate in larger systems to respond to challenges posed by other large systems in their marketplace. The growth of for-profit providers (hospital or physician practices) is now taking advantage of efficiencies and capabilities in managing across multiple markets. In fact, the investment capital that creates national physician enterprises is organizing physician practices at the same level as national insurance companies, national for-profit HMOs, and national hospital management companies.

Other for-profit firms that moved into service delivery include Vencor, MedCath, and HealthSouth. Physician practice management firms have grown signficantly as well. Providing access to capital and management capabilities, practices are owned or managed by contract while physicians have a long-term employment arrangement.

The change in care delivery with increasing managed care continues to emphasize different care modalities with more concentration on both error prevention and standardization (which implies decreased errors), as noted in an editorial in the *New England Journal of Medicine:* "Patients stay in hospitals far fewer days, many surgical procedures that previously required hospitalization are now safely performed in day surgery, there is far more attention to preventive care, many medical practices have been standardized to produce better outcomes and satisfying patients has become an explicit goal."[26]

In a national survey of 400 hospital executives in 1993, it was found that the major priorities facing health care included clinical guidelines, physician-hospital organizations (PHOs), and the number of primary care physicians.[27] The new array of benchmarks to ensure quality—from the perspectives of correct clinical care, error prevention, and patient satisfaction—redefines the parameters of service delivery in a more uniform fashion.

The Buyers Employers actively seek the demonstrated value of health care delivery, which is dictating more services added to the basic set of services. Evaluations of demonstrated value in the context of competitive performance use established quality indicators to compare health plans. HEDIS, which is now part of NCQA and a group of employers and health plans, identifies quality indicators. Of the 60 indicators from HEDIS, 51 focus on process, which is so critical to quality outcomes. Further refinement of the measures likely will be developed as participation in the database grows. Some large employers are creating their own data sets and will have the ability to dictate the premiums they will be willing to pay. Large employers and employer groups are the real drivers of the changes.

Employers and the working population feel the effects of price increases. Employers are actively seeking to restructure plans and reduce their costs. Poverty continues to deepen in this country, often accompanied by a lack of insurance coverage. Social issues that affect the community—domestic violence, education, employment rates, and mental health—also affect costs and the delivery of medical care. Such crises may be partly relieved through pending policy initiatives, but the overall solution lies in community-based care.

MERGING ROLES OF PAYERS AND PROVIDERS

The traditional boundaries between the roles of a payer, acute care provider, and physician provider are disappearing. As payers become providers and providers develop payer products, the line blurs between the clinical and payment systems. IDSs and IDFSs employ physicians and contract with insurance corporations.

Market forces drive integration for a variety of economic reasons, and integration can take many forms, including full-asset mergers and joint ventures. Not all delivery systems that call themselves integrated are integrated. *Modern Healthcare* polled several futurists whose varying observations reflect the evolving nature of the healthcare provider. Some results of the poll were as follows:

- Most of the futurists said they expected that some IDSs will emerge through asset integration, while others will be virtual networks not linked by asset ownership.
- By 2016, large regional networks will be focused on providing a full continuum of care, including long-term care. And the acute care hospital will look different. The demand for inpatient care will shrink by 20 percent to 30 percent, and the most important site for care will be the home, closely followed by the community clinic, according to Jeff Goldsmith, president of a firm that studies trends in health care.
- On the other hand, a futurist who looked at trends in home health care predicted a return to the hospital environment.[28]

Relationships among Payers, Hospitals, and Physicians

These relationships are being continually reshaped, with financial incentives driving varying types of joint arrangements. These types of networks include affiliations, management relationships, joint venture arrangements, and IDSs. Risks and rewards assumed by all players in the entity mean a shared interest in patient management through clinical protocols and utilization, as well as a shared interest in the payment streams. While insurers are more likely to create venture structures, and hospitals and physicians more likely to join together, the options of a three-way capitation arrangement have varying levels of acceptance across the country.

Integration Relationships and Their Benefits

There can be a variety of relationships in integration. As a means of increasing clinical services while reducing costs, integration is an important step for most providers. However, many forms of integration proceed, according to Stephen Shortell, for the sake of creating an integrated system rather than for reasons tied to the market.[29] The following sections list some of the expected benefits of integration for the various relationships:

- hospitals to hospitals
- physicians to physicians
- payers to payers
- hospitals to physicians
- hospitals to payers
- physicians to payers
- traditional and nontraditional channels

Hospitals to Hospitals Among hospitals, there have been a lot of mergers, especially in service areas where there are several acute care providers. In recent years, industry surveys show that hospitals are changing their ownership status, probably in an effort to improve their operating or financial positions.

A review of relationships among acute care health care providers shows that the oft-predicted mergers, including those resulting in closings, have led to consolidation in the hospital industry. In 1990, 43 percent of executives surveyed by Deloitte and Touche said their hospitals could fail within five years.[30] Hospitals are vulnerable, and they prefer consolidation to failure. Following is a list of some of the benefits of such consolidation:

- potential to reduce excess inpatient capacity by closing unneeded acute care beds
- reduced cost of service by eliminating unnecessary duplication and overhead
- elimination of weaker competitors in the marketplace (by incorporating them and right-sizing the set of services in the community)
- the means for subacute care beds located close to acute care services by converting acute care beds to subacute beds
- improved negotiating position for further integration
- greater geographic service area
- more services for a system than single hospitals are able to provide alone
- increased viability of contracts with managed care payers (who want to contract with one entity and increase the choices)

Many of the announcements of hospital mergers reflect a common vision about the future. However, it is clear that initiated merger discussions do not always result in actual mergers.

Physicians to Physicians Physicians, faced with increasingly complex reimbursement for a broader array of payers, integrate their practices with others so that the complexities of contracting and getting paid are ones that can be handled by a broader management structure than a solo physician. Physicians have banded together for more practice support and more sophisticated approaches to managing overhead. Some of the benefits of physician collaboration include

- common approaches to medical care and common service standards of value
- a broader spectrum of clinical care
- more physicians to share expenses of billing, accounting, contracting, information systems, staff support, and facility development and maintenance
- adaptability for physician management companies that are for-profit or not-for-profit
- increased viability of contracts with managed care providers (who want to contract with one entity and increase customer choices)

Payers to Payers Insurers striving for a broad representation of product lines in the indemnity and prepaid sectors acquire firms in order to enter markets and offer the full spectrum of products that employers want. Benefits of these steps include

- access to different types of contracts or product lines
- access to covered lives
- preempting other payers by starting a company to build strong bases
- more rapid entry into a new product area
- immediate increase in market share
- increased contracting capability based on size of enrollment and numbers of providers
- contracting clout

Hospitals to Physicians Hospitals are becoming primary health care providers by acquiring primary care practices and affiliating with management services organizations (MSOs) and PHOs. Long considered the best way to end physician shortages, starting a primary care panel of physician practices is viewed as a means of getting and securing covered lives. The acquisition of a physician base (to secure admissions and patient flow) often has a price tag associated with it that may not be recovered in the management of the practice. Further, the management of physician practices has shown itself to be extremely costly. One of the largest for-profit physician practice management companies executives noted that a third of the prospect calls are from hospital administrators with physician practices operating in a deficit. Among the benefits of integration are the following:

- Hospitals provide capital and managed care contracting capacity.
- To the extent that payers contract with single entities, integration through foundations, MSOs, PHOs, or other entities that can contractually commit both hospital and physician, can ensure provider or payer presence.
- Integration allows for more alignment of incentives among providers so that hospital and physician move together.
- Physicians receive more access to large system capabilities for human resources management, information systems, financial accounting, and marketing capabilities.
- Integration allows for more coordination of care with common clinical protocols to provide the best clinical care with the least duplication in the best environment with the most continuity.

Hospitals to Payers Some hospitals have explored stronger relationships with payers. The challenge has always been the perception of preferred loyalty to one payer over another and missing the opportunity of payer relationships. For the payers, selective contracting eliminates the choice of providers to offer to employers. Benefits include the following:

- information integration to avoid unnecessary duplication
- better information to determine service features that add value to the covered enrollees
- greater access to capital
- coordination of marketing initiatives for both providers and insurers
- cost controls

Physicians to Payers A barrier for payers being able to get market share is the relative shortage of primary care physicians who would or could contract for more covered lives. In the 1990s, hospitals' demand for primary care physicians also has been a problem for growing managed care plans, whose success relies on capacity in a primary care network. Therefore, some payers have invested heavily in key markets to establish physician care centers that would give them the ability to provide care to their enrollees. Among the benefits of physicians-to-payers integration are the following:

- Physicians have stabilized practices.
- Physicians receive the benefit of having their practices managed and potentially share in the financial rewards of the organization.

- Payers get access to primary care providers.
- Payers have an established infrastructure that allows them to amortize the expenses across many primary care physicians.

Traditional and Nontraditional Channels If the consolidation among providers and payers represents a more formalized set of relationships with the traditional participants in the channel to get and keep customers, then the renewed attention to the community's needs represents the nontraditional channels of getting and keeping customers. In anticipation of reform requiring capitation, commitment to a new paradigm shaped the development of community health care networks. In turn, this integrated network approach was shaped to respond to the geographic area served by the network. Public health indicators, such as epidemiological factors, were the driving focus of a provider's responsibilities to local constituents. The drive for a healthier community became part of the commitments by the providers to demonstrate their tax-exempt status as charitable institutions and to fulfill their stated missions. The outreach efforts to reach culturally diverse populations and those who are not able to obtain traditional services and to shape services to respond to multicultural barriers are all part of the real demonstration of value in nontraditional outreach to customers groups.

Role of Integration to Move toward Market Advantage

This decade's flirtation with health care reform and the buyers' requirements for low cost and provider choice encouraged free market enterprise to move toward consolidation. Consolidation benefits include decreasing costs to achieve a more competitive position or enhance market position. Increasingly, physicians, hospitals, and non-acute care providers are players in this consolidation. The proposed health reform payment system under capitation and the anticipated growth as a payment system provides incentives to manage health status compared to managing disease or injury incidence. While managing long-term outcomes in clinical care, managing short-term relationships remains a necessary and important factor in establishing health care networks.

CONCLUSION

To respond to the enormous changes faced by the health care industry today, organizations must be flexible, informed, and strategically prepared. A planning process can provide direction, showing how to improve the delivery of care while maximizing reimbursement. Changes in network structure, provider relationships, reimbursement, and economic incentives require that organizations take advantages of opportunities, work with multiple contingencies, achieve self-knowledge, and move quickly and intelligently. A plan that reflects the vision and values of the organization and is aligned with the currents in the marketplace is essential for any organization moving into the future.

References

1. VHA, Inc., *Market Forces and Critical Success Factors: An Executive Report for VHA Health Care Organizations* (Irving, Tex.: VHA, Inc., 1994), p. 15.

2. Paul Starr, *The Logic of Health Care Reform* (Grand Rounds Press, 1992), pp. 73-74.

3. Theodore Levitt, *Thinking About Management* (New York: The Free Press, 1991), p. 94.

4. Stan Davis, *The Monster Under the Bed* (New York: Simon & Schuster, 1994), p. 111.

5. Levitt, *Thinking About Management,* pp. 93–94.

6. Lance Heineccius, "Columbia/HCA: A National Profile," *Washington State Hospital Association* (Dec. 1, 1995): 18.

7. Quoted in Terese Hudson, "Mapping the Future: 'The Dartmouth Atlas,'" *Hospitals & Health Networks* 70, no. 7 (Apr. 5, 1996): 26.

8. Peter F. Drucker, *Managing for the Future: The 1990s and Beyond* (New York: Dutton, 1992), p. 20.

9. *New York Times* (July 30, 1996): 1.

10. *New York Times* (July 30, 1996); and interview with Nancy Dubler, Director of the Division of Bioethics, Montefiore Medical Center, New York, N.Y.

11. Levitt, *Thinking About Management,* pp. 94-95.

12. Nancy Dubler, presentation to the Metropolitan Boston Society for Health Care Planning and Marketing, 1993.

13. Paul Starr, *The Social Transformation of American Medicine* (Boston: Basic Books, 1982), p. 278.

14. Robert G. Shouldice and Katherine H. Shouldice, *Medical Group Practice and Health Maintenance Organizations* (Washington, D.C.: Information Resources Press, 1978), p. 38.

15. Starr, *The Social Transformation,* p. 352.

16. Ibid., p. 298.

17. Ibid., p. 313.

18. Ibid., p. 339.

19. Ibid., p. 381.

20. Jeff C. Goldsmith, *Can Hospitals Survive?* (Homewood, Ill.: Dow Jones Irwin, 1981), pp. 30-31.

21. U.S. Department of Health Education and Welfare, *A Report to the President on Medical Care Prices* (Washington, D.C.: U.S. Government Printing Office, 1967), pp. 4-5.

22. Starr, *The Social Transformation,* p. 380.

23. A. S. Relman, "The New Medical-Industrial Complex." *New England Journal of Medicine* 303 (1980): 936-70.

24. E. Marszalek-Gaucherand and R. J. Coffey, *Transforming Health Care Organizations: How to Achieve and Sustain Organizational Excellence* (San Francisco: Jossey-Bass, 1990), p. 117.

25. *Modern Healthcare* (Aug. 26, 1996).

26. Jerome Kassirer, "Managed Care and the Morality of the Marketplace," *New England Journal of Medicine* (July 6, 1996): 50.

27. Frank Cerne, "Prepared for Uncertainty?" *Hospitals & Health Networks* 67, no. 16 (Aug. 20, 1993): 22-25.

28. *Modern Healthcare* (Aug. 26, 1996).

29. "The Big Picture: A Conversation with Stephen Shortell," *Health Systems Review* (July/Aug. 1996): 25-27.

30. *Modern Healthcare* (June 1990).

2

The Strategic Plan Development Process

Planning is everything. The plan is nothing.

—*Dwight D. Eisenhower*

Executive Summary

Planning has changed from a centralized activity to a decentralized one. This evolution has been, in many ways, necessary, to take advantage of such competitive strategies as quality improvement and enhancements in reengineering.

A strategic plan relies on shared values and a common vision as much as on the analytic information that was once the focus of strategic planning. Thus, strategic plan development must be viewed as a means of charting the organization's future. The steps in an effective strategic plan development process reflect the organization's vision and values and culminate in development of an action plan. However, the organization must be wary of such pitfalls as lack of employee and management commitment, cumbersome processes, and inflexible planning systems that can prevent a strategic plan from succeeding.

INTRODUCTION

Planning is the act of integrating an entity's mission statement and goals, taking marketplace and environmental realities into account to reach the goals within the bounds of the mission statement. A plan, on the other hand, contains the written results of the planning function. Planning is an active process, the plan is a guide to implement that action. As long as management is committed to the plan, planning sets the sights of the organization. The three components of strategic planning are

- *consensus:* the general agreement among involved parties about the strategic challenges, opportunities, and directions
- *vision:* the picture of what the organization is becoming
- *analytical information:* knowledge about marketplace and the organization's performance

After the plan is completed, changes in the internal or external environment may require adjustments. Further, the strategy development process requires the resolution of short- and long-term challenges.

Strategic directions reflect the actions taken to achieve the vision for the organization and help the organization navigate among the external circumstances to achieve its chosen direction. If the management agenda includes the plan's stated activities, then the plan is more than just a report gathering dust on a shelf. Whit Spaulding, former president of the Society for Healthcare Planning and Marketing, sees planning as a way to differentiate between the document and the action: "Planning . . . [is] documents to show population projections, market share trends, age profile of physicians and other boring data. The real plan might be . . . Our anesthesia department is lousy so we'll force the chief into early retirement and hire the new professor from the University to turn our anesthesia program into a first class operation."[1]

This chapter reviews the steps of a strategic plan development process and the implications for plan implementation. It also discusses the difficulties involved in developing a strategic plan.

STEPS IN THE PROCESS OF STRATEGIC PLAN DEVELOPMENT

Strategic plan development is a process that builds a consensus, focuses on the future, engages organizational commitment, and identifies actions to make the resulting plan operational. The process incorporates strategic inputs on the environment, relevant updates on industry changes, reflection on the organization's position, and definition of the vision and values. This process answers the following questions:

- *Who are we?* This question calls for a review of the organization's mission and current situation.
- *What is happening around us?* This question includes what is happening on an industry-wide basis and in the regional marketplace.

- *Where are we going?* This question calls for vision formulation about what the organization may do, given the context of the industry, regional situation, and organizational resources and position.
- *How will we get there?* This question focuses on the development of strategies to achieve the vision as well as the action plan that drives the process of implementation.

Figure 2-1 summarizes the steps inherent in the plan development process. Each step is critical to the future of a health care organization.

Step 1. Review Prior Plans and Planning Processes

The first step is to audit the prior strategic plans and determine what actions were committed to. Even if the management team has changed, it is unlikely that the board and the medical staff have changed so much that prior promises of strategy have been forgotten. The players from the prior planning process still live with some expectation that identified directions of the prior plan will continue to be pursued. Therefore, a review of prior plans and the subsequent updates and reports to the planning committee can bring closure to prior plan commitments and set the stage for the next round of challenges. Lack of continuity can cause duplication, confusion, and frustration, as can be seen by the following true story:

In one community hospital, a new management team initiated a strategy development process a year after a previous strategic plan had been developed. The new process included quantitative input and gave comprehensive recommendations. Six months after the completion of the plan, the board requested management to update the recommendations from the *original* plan and meet with the consultant to become familiar with those recommendations. The planning office initiated work with the first consultants to review the context for their recommendations. If a review, update, and modification of the first plan's directions had been incorporated into the subsequent planning process, management would not have faced such a dilemma.

The review of prior plans calls for review of the problems confronting the organization at that time, the supporting data and reasons, and the recommended actions to resolve those challenges. Thus, the review should include

- *A review of every recommended action:* Recommendations may or may not have solved the organization's perceived problems at the time of the planning process. They also may have been based on temporarily apparent problems or solutions. For example, a

FIGURE 2-1. Plan Development Chart

Step 1. Review Prior Plans and Planning Processes

The review of earlier strategic plans and planning processes introduces suggestions about what works and does not work in the organization. These lessons include the role of leadership, employee and affiliated physician alignment, previous priorities and historical drivers for those priorities, and the reaction to the subsequent implementation or nonimplementation.

Step 2. Prepare an Agenda for the Planning Process

The preparation of the agenda that will occupy committee and management attention is important so that the participants will know what to expect throughout the process.

Step 3. Do an Environmental Analysis

This component reviews overall changes in regulation, payment patterns, and integration criteria, as well as innovations. Review of local, regional, and national markets and trends is useful in considering both organizational initiatives and collaboration opportunities.

Step 4. Conduct a Values Clarification

Values clarification reflects both currently held values and those that are needed for the evolving organization in the future. The leaders take stock about the principles they share and need in the future to achieve the vision.

Step 5. Articulate the Vision Statement

The future picture of what the organization will look like is the vision statement. The vision statement defines the reason for an organization's existence, the role the organization is going to play in its marketplace, and what it will look like.

Step 6. Clarify the Organization's Strategy Options

The strategy options are the functional means of achieving the vision through understanding how to prepare for the future in the following categorical ways:

- payer assessment/position
- physician network assessment/position
- organizational performance/capability
- financial capability/now and potential
- merger and alliance position
- getting and keeping customers

Step 7. Develop an Action Plan

The range of strategy options will suggest immediate and long-term actions. The importance of establishing priorities and clarifying expected actions and outcomes are management's guide to its work in moving ahead to realize the vision of the organization.

hospital dealing with a declining inpatient market share would not have that problem solved by the development of a minor care walk-in service, a solution typically used to add acute patient volume to empty beds.

- *A review of the supporting data for reasons for actions:* The data underlying recommendations must be reviewed and updated continuously. For example, a hospital relying on publicly available information may find indications that some area providers plan to establish primary care provider sites in outlying areas—an action that may threaten established practices. To rely on these data, without some sort of independent verification that the planned action is in fact likely to occur, may lead the planning organization to make decisions based on misinformation. What are the actual data that supported a recommendation? What are the reasons for an action?

- *A review of the currency of the supporting data/reasons:* The data that lead to recommended actions can quickly become outdated. If the data indicators no longer hold true, or if there have been significant changes in the data categories, expectations for the conclusion of that recommended action would be altered. For example, projected growth of a residential area has been reversed due to a downward turn for the major area employer. What is the source of the data? What is the most recent update of the data supporting the actions? How current are those same reasons? Are the data still applicable? Are the same threats to growth or stability still there?

- *A review of the status on recommended action:* The recommended action may have been a single management intervention or a new approach that would affect operations. Has that action been carried out? Is it still in process of being developed or implemented? Has it been determined to be unfeasible or to create problems elsewhere in the organization? The status of each prior recommended action is important to the management so that it can strategically respond.

- *Expected versus actual outcome of the recommended action:* The recommended action was intended to solve a problem. What was the expected outcome of the action? What is the actual outcome of the recommended action (if put into place)? How successful was this initiative? If not successful, what was missing? Recommended actions probably projected some return, whether it was in cost savings, clinical service quality, operational efficiency, financial or volume gain, or differentiation from competition. Comparison of the actual and expected outcomes might predict the success of the planning process in the next iteration of planning.

- *Rate the validity today of this recommended action:* The recommended action may continue to be relevant and worth current action. If however, after review, it is no longer valid, then such an amendment to the recommended action is noted.

The previous planning processes should be reviewed in order to know how the organization and its leadership made prior strategic commitments. Even with a new management team, there are lessons to be learned from previous successes and failures. Understanding how previous decisions have or have not been productive, relevant, or efficient helps to evaluate the process by which those decisions were made. Prior planning processes should be reviewed in order to

- Assess the relevant drivers of the strategic recommendations that may contribute to the current plan development.
- Bring closure to prior plans by updating the planning committee.
- Review the lessons learned about participation and leadership in both the plan development and implementation.

Step 2. Prepare an Agenda for the Planning Process

The agenda for the planning process is threefold: leadership preparation, participant preparation, and agenda construction.

Preparing Leadership   The strategic planning process requires leadership commitment to both the process and the implementation. Strategy development requires risk-oriented management behavior and the organizational leader's commitment to process and to bringing the organization along.

The leader of the organization's commitment to the strategic planning process is the driving factor for its success. He or she must sign off on it, stand behind the implementation, and motivate the relevant parties to move ahead. Current management and leadership literature shows the importance of visionary leadership demonstrated by the leader of the organization. There may be compelling problems to solve on an immediate basis before initiating a strategic planning process.

The organization of the leadership process includes configuring the planning committee that will oversee the development and implementation of the plan. Committee representation includes members of the management team, medical staff, and board. There may be others needed for the committee as well. The committee's exact charge is identified in the organization's bylaws. There are two approaches to developing a strategic plan oversight group:

1. *Use a standing committee of the board:* That committee includes managers, board members, and physicians. The board's formal processes for establishing membership terms and the committee purpose make it a regular part of organizational life.
2. *Use a short-term task force:* This type of appointed task force operates for a limited time. The group meets for the sole purpose of developing the strategic plan and reports to the president. Task force membership includes those most affected by the initiatives and whose participation is critical to the success of the organization. Members are selected for their ability to represent the issues and concerns of the group they represent and their ability to influence the direction of the organization among their peers. Members may include both informal and formal leaders.

The planning committee oversees and governs the planning activity of the organization. It operates as a subcommittee of the board of trustees. The advantage of this structure is that it serves in a continuing role to oversee the strategic planning process and the implementation.

Preparing Participants Preparation for the planning process should be based on short interviews or small focus groups with the players. This preparation is a great way to discuss current problems and needs as well as identify organization values. The preparation of the planning agenda should ensure that specific issues are addressed. It is important to ask the participants about their perspectives on critical issues of strategic importance, including both internal and external elements and positive and negative issues. That is not the same as the market research, which is addressed in chapter 3. It is an effort to gain perspective and understand expectations.

Three major issues that should be explored in a preplanning interview process with key planning participants (both past and current) are as follows:

1. *Reaction to the prior planning activities:* Key issues identified in the interviews will need to be addressed in the formation of the planning process. If there were adverse reactions to prior planning processes, then those processes must be reconciled with the needs of the players. The organization that conducted a strategy development process, without having considered the interests of a key customer group, would need to explain that omission and to make sure to include it in future information gathering. Employers' priorities as they manage benefits and consumers' priorities as they buy insurance are important when a health care provider decides in which payer networks to participate. The lack of information that results in not participating in relevant networks may lead to a loss of enrollees.

2. *Expectations and goals for the upcoming planning process:* The identification of participants' goals for the planning process is another means of formulating the agenda for strategic planning. In addition, this preparation provides a basis for understanding the expected outcomes and shaping the group's education before, during, and after the planning process.

3. *The perception of the organization:* The participants' understanding of the key external players helps to identify outstanding issues and to formulate the introduction to the planning process. This information helps to clarify or set the expectations at the beginning of the process.

Developing the Committee Agenda The expected outcome of the planning committee's work should be determined before the agenda and meeting forums are planned. The functional tasks of establishing a planning process include the development of meeting planning tactics, such as establishing a schedule and location, and decisions about the environment in which the committee will function. A thoughtful, focused discussion, with relevant presentations and suggested implications, directions, and shape, will help shape the committee's agenda. The planning schedule should provide focus and help establish priorities for the committee agenda:

- decide who the facilitator will be for the following activities:
  —values discussion
  —data collection and presentation
  —vision interpretation
  —strategic options
- staff preparation of meeting times and logistics
  —assessment of prior planning activities
  —updates for the current planning process
  —scope of presentations and discussion in committee
- review of planning data

The committee composition assumes that the facilitator is not also a participant. The facilitator's sole responsibility is to guide the discussion. Using one of the participants as a facilitator may hinder his or her ability to contribute opinions and insights. More information pertaining to teams is included in chapter 4.

At the senior level, there are both working familiarity with the vision and the ability to work collaboratively with other members of the leadership group. Plan directions and conclusions are drawn from many discussions, which are sorted and prioritized in keeping with the company's vision. Support staff or consultants collect and analyze strategic information and present it in a compelling fashion to facilitate discussion and decision making.

A consultant frees management to participate in plan development and to express its biases. The consultant that leads or facilitates the process coordinates with the assigned senior manager and the CEO. Depending on the needs of the strategic planning process, different consultants may be engaged for different parts of the work. For example, for the organization with multiple needs that include development of values and vision statements, there may be a need for a more process-oriented consultant instead of an analytic strategy consultant.

A consultant may be used to manage the process, generate the strategic options, and offer second opinions. The last role is a useful way to test the viability of the strategic directions by garnering a relatively independent reaction toward options. A planning team benefits from a consultant challenging its conclusions and assumptions. As with using a facilitator who is not part of the process, the consultant is not torn among the requirements of facilitating, participating, and stating his or her own opinions.

The specific roles in which a consultant could be helpful include providing the industry update, facilitating the values summary and formulating the future values statement, and facilitating the formulation of the vision statement. Some consultants report being engaged as a sounding board or second opinion on technical support, process direction, and strategic conclusions. Consultants may also play the following roles:

- advocates or champions to orchestrate the process and keep the organizations moving
- trainers to educate the staff on the planning process, the timetable, and expected results
- facilitators to deal with small-group process issues, including group norms to allow challenges or confrontations
- coaches or content experts to counsel the planning group on best practices and to supervise technical analysis and presentation
- strategists to be current on available strategies for the organization
- "lightning rods" to put for controversial points and get reactions

Step 3. Do an Environmental Analysis

An environmental analysis is important in assessing national trends, regional trends, and local opportunities. This analysis calls for examining both business trends and health care–related trends. Expert resources are often found essential to formulating the final conclusions about the environmental trends and beliefs about how the national and regional markets appear.

The variation in markets across the country makes it difficult to apply solutions from other markets to local problems because they lack a common framework. As a result, education of the planning team is very important. The content would include the scope of changes on a national and regional basis. The benefit of this type of education would be to broaden the expectations of the possibilities for both the market and the organization. An environmental analysis would look at such factors as

- *Industry drivers:* The industry drivers on a national basis are critical to looking at the larger framework of the industry. The regional marketplace analysis and conclusions summarize the environment of the organization. Industry drivers have a profound impact, for example, on the potential for a national health care policy and Medicare and Medicaid reform. Accordingly, the summation of the internal strengths and weaknesses and the external strengths and opportunities provide strategic input into the strategy assessment and conclusion for the organization.
- *New players in the market:* New providers and payers have an impact on the health care industry. The new players could enter any market. If there is any type of new entrant into a local market, that must be considered when assessing the industry. The development of the industry trends shapes the values, vision, and development of strategic options for an organization.
- *Change in industry boundaries:* Even the definition of what industry is to be analyzed is often uncertain. In this time of immense change in organizations, each organization in a transformation moves into new industries. The development of an information technology to support more complex organization means a move into information systems. One analyst has even identified a paradoxical "death of competition": "As traditional industry boundaries erode around us, companies often unexpectedly find themselves in fierce competition with unlikely rivals. . . . Is Wal-Mart a retailer, a wholesaler, or an information services and logistics company?"[2]
- *Strategic inputs:* Conclusions about the industry, the dominant paradigms, and local markets are drawn from a detailed assessment of the strategic inputs, which are identified in chapter 3. The health care industry seems torn between preparing for a model of integration and a model of market response based on the managed care penetration. The intent of integration has many benefits, and many organizations are developing integrated delivery systems.
- *Degree of managed care penetration:* Many organizations are developing responses to greater levels of managed care, even those not necessarily paid on a fully capitated basis. However, there are two models of progression in the business life cycle of the marketplace,

based on the managed care market characteristics, and the subsequent response of the consumers' attraction mechanisms. Those models are reviewed in chapter 3, and the selection of an ultimate strategy lies in identifying the greatest value added to the future of the organization, based on the marketplace challenges.

Step 4. Conduct Values Clarification

An organization's values are how its members identify what is important as the organization evolves to become the shape foreseen in the vision. The clarification and articulation of company values have become more widespread across all industries as a means of unifying the workforce. Since the 1980s, business pressure has focused on restructuring workforce accountability and authority to put information in the hands of those closest to the customer, empowering them to make decisions. Subsequently, the employees' motivation and alignment with the organization's vision provide the most effective service. The corporate values guide the way the work will be done and ways in which the organization makes decisions, allocates resources, and conducts business.

Burt Nanus describes the role of the values in the organization: "Values are the principles or standards that help people decide what is worthwhile or desirable. They are abstract ideas that embody notions of what truly matters or should matter, in the performance of an organization and in the ways an organization satisfies its responsibilities to its constituencies—workers, customers, investors and the rest of society."[3] The process of articulating the values may suggest a change in values. With the industry review, the need for change may underscore the need to change the values. The values that an organization has held may be different from the values that the organization will hold. A traditional organization rewarded longevity of service and loyalty to the administration. However, the environment and the goals may require results-oriented innovation and entrepreneurial activities. The revised values statement will assist in pointing out the ways in which new behaviors are supported and motivated.

Identifying the Organization's Values There are several ways to identify an organization's current values and clarify the values needed for the organization to make the changes needed for the future. The steps of asking about current values and anticipated values are different. The techniques to identify the values are as follows:

- Interview a collection of senior and middle managers, as well as experienced staff.
- Conduct employee-focus groups among various groups of employees, including management.
- Conduct a survey among employees.

The same audience may be asked to articulate the relevant values to accomplish the stated vision or expected outcome. Subsequently, the audience (interviewees, focus group participants, or survey participants) would identify the values that the changes would represent.

Conducting a Value Audit One means of assessing the values is to conduct a value audit, which includes the following steps:

- List the published or documented values of the organization.
- List the actual values practiced by the organization.
- List the values hindering the organization (either personal or organizational) and note the disparities.
- Create a list of value statements that will solidify and provide a foundation for the values that will most support the business objectives.[4]

Such steps in identifying the explicit and implicit values serve as a starting point in declaring what values are the most important. In fact, the values that are most closely held may be different from the ones needed to achieve the organization's desired or stated visions. The development of a values statement that mirrors the vision statement is an essential part of the plan.

Articulating the Organization's Values One technique suggested for a group to articulate organizational values is for the planning committee to review their perspective of the organization's values. Specifically, the values scan has five elements:

1. the personal values of the planning team
2. the values of the organization as a whole
3. the organization's operational philosophy
4. the organization's culture
5. the organization's stakeholders[5]

This approach is particularly useful in separating the values of those on the planning committee and the values seen for the organization. Because the committee includes the organization's leadership, its viewpoint for its own participation and the committee's view of the organization are likely to be similar to information gathered from others.

Although the above-described process takes into account the value orientation of the planning committee, the staff's values should be incorporated and recognized. That information would be shared with the planning committee to integrate into the organization's values review. Gathering information from staff groups may take the form of research through surveys of key groups (such as employees and physicians), focus groups, or multiple interviews.

Step 5. Articulate the Vision Statement

An organization's vision is the image of what it—and its core purposes—will be in the future. Around that vision, the strategic plan establishes a timeline of objectives and deliverables. The vision serves to bring together the employees, management, and affiliated physicians around the central focus of where the organization is going. United by a central direction, structural conflicts become clearer in their solutions. *The Portable MBA* tells this story: "Once Kodak declared their own strategic intent to remain a world leader in imaging . . . debates inside the company on whether chemical imaging was superior to electronic imaging or vice versa, subsided. The focus shifted to creating new hybrids—products and services that creatively combined both chemical and electronic capability."[6]

Relating the Vision to Historical Statements The vision is related to other historical statements. The historical statement is the mission statement that most nonprofit organizations have. The mission statement denotes the purpose of the organization, although it tends to be broad and encompass so many commitments that it has no strategic value in setting direction. It is, however, the focus of the organization, around which services have been developed, donations have been solicited, and the charitable nature of the organization has been established.

The values already discussed reveal how the organization conducts itself with its constituent groups. It also clarifies how the organization will achieve the vision and the manner in which it will conduct itself in management activities and decisions. The initial vision of the organization is developed and guides the consideration of the strategy process. Although based on a practical plan, there may be a need for reconsideration for the vision, depending on the willingness to make commitments to the actions that would achieve the vision. For example, an organization that wishes to assume a preeminent place in the marketplace but has neither the capital nor expertise to attain that position would likely seek an affiliation with another organization to move in that direction.

Relating the Vision to Future Statements The vision will be able to incorporate some of the possibilities laid out in the examples from other components. This framework emboldens the group to create a future vision that is daring and productive, while at the same time the mission statement ensures consistency with the founding purpose. The vision directs an organization toward the future while still allowing enough flexibility to respond to local and immediate challenges. Henry Mintzberg, an expert on strategic planning, has written, "The visionary approach is a more flexible way to deal with an uncertain world. Vision sets the broad outlines of a strategy, while leaving the specific details to be worked out. In other words, the broad perspective may be deliberate but the specific positions can emerge. So when the unexpected happens, assuming the vision is sufficiently robust, the organization can adapt—it learns. Certain change is thus easily accommodated."[7]

Developing a Vision Statement Because vision development suggests that organizations need to think ahead, it is easiest to start with concrete ideas in the near term for review, discussions, and further consideration. Many experts comment that the best means to achieve a common vision is to develop one's own vision and, drawing from common interests, develop a corporate vision. Some comment that the organization has a vision that is based on insight from key formal and informal leaders, such as Henry Ford's belief that anyone could own a car. Strong leadership in an organization often indicates that vision is based on the direction of the CEO and shared by the management team. An example of this is the early success of Apple Computers, where the leadership (Steven Jobs and Steve Wozniak) believed that the computer could empower people.

In an article in *Modern Healthcare,* David Burda describes a vision statement designed for a merger between two medical centers in Maine:

> When Maine Medical Center Foundation was formed as the governing body for the merger of Maine Medical Center and Brighton Medical Center, it was based on a vision for the merger. Each organization would keep the respective CEO and a new CEO would be recruited to govern the Foundation. The merger was formed to gain control of the market share and reduce costs, leading to economic efficiency, since the Foundation now contains 68% of Portland's staff beds. The vision of the merger is: "The hospitals will be committed to reducing the overall cost of health care in the community, by eliminating all possible duplication of clinical and administrative services. Resultant savings in operating and capital costs will accrue to the benefit of the community."[8]

The challenge to developing a vision statement is to set the context in a broad and opportunity-oriented way, allowing participants in the strategy process to bring to the table their own creative solutions to make the vision operational.

The vision statement, reviewed by the planning committee, is also shared with the board, medical staff leadership group, and other key leadership groups to get input. The sharing of the vision statement with others is part of growing a future vision together. The way in which the vision is communicated is key and will embody the value of communication and employee buy-in. It is a great opportunity to work with employees in a new way. The vision statement will be finalized at the leadership level for consistency with the organization's activities and initiatives, relevance to the marketplace, and the scope of activities.

Step 6. Clarify the Organization's Strategy Options

There are several straightforward ways of clarifying the strategic directions for an organization. Partly, it may be the formal means of articulating what others have been saying for some time. From extensive interviews and sets of discussion, subjects will emerge that are issues or opportunities for the organization. Henry Mintzberg has identified three means of delivering strategic directions:

1. *Codify the strategy:* Clarify and express the strategy in terms sufficiently clear to make it operational, so that its consequences can be worked out in detail. This is affirming the consensus and commitment as it occurs. The planning process has been described as "the decisions just made are symbolically strewn about the table"; the planner puts them together and converts them from general thoughts to specific directives.
2. *Elaborate the strategy:* Develop sub-strategies at the corporate, business, or functional levels, otherwise noted as a "timed sequence of conditional moves in resource deployment." While this is a more formalized approach, it is relevant for programming and implementing although not for the formulation of strategy.
3. *Convert the elaborated strategy:* This is the determination of the consequences of the programmatic changes on the routine operations of the organization—performance control. Objectives are restated and budgets reworked, policies and standard operating procedures reconsidered, to take into account the consequences of the specific changes in action. That can only take place after strategic learning has been completed and strategic thinking has converged on appropriate patterns.[9]

Each of the components of strategic learning has likely generated ideas and decisions with a wide variety of timelines associated with them. Although the adoption of a vision allows flexibility in considering what an organization will become, the imperative to achieve it may tempt a management team to set a time frame for strategic change that is too short, such as total accomplishment within 18 months. That short of a time frame for achieving the organization's strategies may limit day-to-day management's ability to respond to the organization's changes. The time frame for forming the strategic directions should be adequate to accomplish the constituent tasks. Some goals might require an outlook stretching 5 to 10 years or more.

Recommitment to the Mission Commitment to the historical mission of the organization needs to be revisited. Developing the strategic future of the organization may have a completely different vision and plan but still should parallel the mission statement. For example, the realities of the marketplace, based on strategic inputs, showed Children's Hospital in Baltimore the requirements for change for them to continue as a facility: "If all goes according to plan, the 86-year-old Children's Hospital will open a 114-bed long-term care facility by 1997 and will build an assisted living home, adult day care facility, and other types of care for the elderly on its 45-acre property during the next five years. The long-term care project is one of the ways that the facility plans to make a comeback after four years of losses and a dwindling occupancy rate in its 76-bed acute care unit."[10]

It is important to ensure that the directions set in the planning process are achievable. Admittedly, many organizations face unique challenges in their own marketplace and may have issues that require responses that are outside of the following framework. The strategy framework is only intended as a guide. The basic components are as follows:

- payer assessment and position
- physician network assessment and position
- organizational performance and capability
- current and potential financial capability
- merger or alliance position
- getting and keeping customers

Payer Assessment and Position Revenue sources drive all businesses. Over the years, the payers for health care services have been changing their terms of payment and criteria for doing business. Medicare, as a dominant player, has priorities that have dictated most of what makes up acute care service delivery. Most hospitals' program decisions are founded on Medicare reimbursement regulations. For example, subacute care services located in hospitals grew when the reimbursement opportunity was presented both to develop a step-down level of care and to be reimbursed on the basis of cost. If Medicare changes its criteria for payment, the growth of subacute services may slow. If global payments become a large portion of reimbursement to a health care system, without penalizing both acute and subacute stages of care delivery, then they may become a cost-efficient means of care management.

Because the history of health care service development has been shaped by what the payers would allow, the change in payment mechanism has facilitated a change in the shape of service delivery. Therefore, the first and foremost strategic position is managing the payers—responding to them and negotiating with them. Taking a position with the payers and establishing a payer platform for minimum and preferred contracting mechanisms is an essential step for financial stability and the shape of the allowable and reimbursable service configuration. It is essential to involve the clinicians and their requirements for shaping the payer platform and then to develop tools to jointly manage the patient base.

The position of the payer contracts makes or breaks the health care delivery system's financial position. Short-term contracts mean an organization will have a short-lived financial position, where the payment terms are secure only as long as the contract period. Contracts with no-cause termination clauses also mean a potentially short-lived financially secure position. Therefore, the strategic future has much to do with the assessment of the current payers in the market, the organization's payer position, and the payers' response to that position. Finally, there will be choices to make about keeping or changing the relationship with the payers.

Positioning oneself in the marketplace always has been important, but positioning decisions are not easy. Payers choose providers based on a wide range of criteria, including price, services offered, customer needs, and continued contentment. If a provider wants to stay stable or, preferably, to grow, it must consider all these factors.

The role of the payer is more important when one is not relying on a cost-based reimbursement system. Payers will selectively contract with specific providers, using clinical and cost criteria for selection. Because the patient (customer) selects insurance based on the available payers (and the cost of the premium and copayments), the payer rises in importance as a means of securing a large volume of patients. That challenge demands a strategy regarding payer position.

Even the provider in an apparently isolated service area faces competition from peripheral providers. Therefore, when negotiating new contracts, it is important to clarify the current volume in specific employer accounts and how the payer expects to hold or increase covered lives. The market with several providers means that exclusive contracting may transfer volume from other providers and provide new volume. The stabilizing of current volume involves keeping a payer from moving covered lives to other providers.

An assessment also may be made of payer and provider behavior in another state or in another system. A current review of the nation's similar or more advanced state or urban markets, based on the level of managed care activity, is easily obtained. An organization may use the data from more progressive states or progressive organizations for their learning potential. Payers and providers in more mature markets who have more experience with the market changes are candidates to watch. In addition, the more mature markets also provide models for potential scenario development (as discussed in chapter 3), as an organization compares its market or seeks models against which to compare its current and anticipated performance.

The financial requirements for the acute care facility must be determined, including the extent of marginal pricing that would be used for incremental volume. However, in considering these variables for a contracting platform, extensive discounts or low prices given to a payer for what seems like new volume may be "switched volume" rather than "new volume." Switched volume occurs when people already utilizing the health care system move to another payer for the low rates. New volume comes from attracting new people into the system. Another challenge to low pricing for new volume is that the contracting payment system will only pay less as time progresses and other payers demand parity in contracting.

The extent to which a medical community can develop a contracting vehicle with hospitals and physicians eases contracting for payers and unites the medical community (acute care providers, primary care physicians, and specialists). A position on contract vehicle is an important strategic decision for many providers, both physicians and acute care providers. In any case, decisions by each type of provider are best made in consideration of the other clinical "partners," such as a decision about contracting vehicles in the future.

The health care provider should assess its cost and value position compared to industry standards and state and regional players. The health care organization that demonstrates lower cost or cost efficiency on an encounter basis has an advantage in the industry for the purposes of contracting. The payers demonstrating value through charge discounts are not differentiating between the high- and low-cost providers. However, the payers developing more in-depth relationships, based on case rates or diagnosis-related group (DRG) rates, will appreciate the lower cost per discharge. Similarly, the length-of-stay efficiency, again demonstrated on a case mix adjusted basis compared to industry, state, and regional players, offers another area to demonstrate value. The payers demonstrating value through per diem contract rates will not take advantage of the provider of a shorter length of stay. The payer relationship that relies on length-of-stay efficiency should have contract terms rewarding the provider showing better cost efficiency.

The opportunity to become repositioned for better payer participation will affect the entire system of care. The pricing strategy, the delivery efficiency and protocols, and the range of services available are all affected. Demonstrable value is also based on the physician network, which is discussed later in this chapter. A strategic plan either will address these key areas or call for the specifics to address these areas. It has been said that the gain of market power necessary to succeed in the 1990s is the result of favorable negotiation of terms between the payer and provider.

If a payer platform is found acceptable, the associated tactics might look like any of the following:

- Establish a provider vehicle for both physicians and the acute care provider.
- Set payment terms that are more favorable for exclusive contracts.
- Set payment terms that are more favorable for longer term contracts.
- Contract so that there is participation in major payer networks on favorable terms.
- Increase primary care access by increasing the primary care network to appeal to new and growing payers who need the capacity.
- Quantify goals of cost and value to secure and retain managed care contracts with demonstrated quality factors.
- Determine capitation payments with assistance of actuarial experts.
- Work with the full provider community to capture capitation payments.
- Decrease costs in service delivery and increase efficiencies in service delivery to improve contracting position and get economic stability with payers.

Physician Network Assessment and Position The economic integration of acute care providers and physicians is a critical component of a health care organization. Physicians can develop a network with the support of a payer or acute care provider. Physicians working together represent a critical mass both in terms of having greater leverage with payers and in sharing the overhead costs of developing an expensive infrastructure for their practices. To have a future, every health care organization must have a position on how to work with physicians, whether it is a formal or informal association, while physician organizations determine their relationships with each other and with new members. Contracting issues and access to a primary care physician network ensure service delivery access.

Any organization has to have a position on working with physicians. For a physician group, unless the group is already large enough to independently secure a health care organization or provider contracts for a market area, the group must grow. The emphasis on the physicians' relationships with health care organizations took formal hold in the 1980s with the consideration of "physician bonding" (the practice of contractually tying members of the medical staff to hospitals). Together, physicians and health care delivery organizations can work together to contract with providers and work toward providing a seamless, low-cost system of care.

In the last 10 years, physician bonding has focused on securing procedural work, ancillary referrals, and admissions. Recently physician bonding is moving toward a more secure means of physician engagement through a corporate affiliation, employment, and practice management. Many providers view a physician network connected through employment as putting the integration where it belongs and as a means of creating a strong affiliation to align incentives.

When forming physician networks, the organization and the providers must consider the allocation of costs—whether creating a new network or acquiring an existing one. The organization also must consider the fit between the physicians and the organization, and whether they share visions and values.

Establishing or expanding a primary care network may be accomplished by establishing new physician practices or acquiring existing practices (the "make or buy" scenario). Starting a provider-sponsored network requires hiring physicians, buying or leasing space (and doing the necessary renovations), and putting practice management into place. Making new practices takes longer and requires more front-end capital than buying existing practices.

In contrast, establishing contracts with existing providers allows more rapid entry into the market. It also may require a transition plan to achieve financial efficiencies of group management—centralized billing, scheduling systems, and financial reporting—not to mention a central location. Practices that are located centrally are able to take advantage of using common support systems to get efficiencies in overhead and staffing. In contrast, small practices carry overhead that cannot be shared, such as the building, equipment, computers, and telephone systems. Small group practices or solo practices duplicate office expenses. In a centrally located practice, such expenses could be allocated among more practitioners.

Aligning the medical staff is necessary to achieve a successful physician program outcome. Aligning physicians depends on shared values and vision. The following list contains assumptions, which, if shared by physician leadership, can result in successful collaborative outcomes:

- The shape of the future is better if the physicians, or provider and physicians, contract together as one entity.
- The primary care providers should be expanded in concert with existing physicians.
- The collaborative needs to stabilize the specialists through inclusion in payer contracting and to augment gaps in the specialty services.
- The payer contracting position will be strengthened with more primary care physician access; highly productive physicians; and a low-cost, but high-value, delivery system that will allow more covered lives into the contracting system.
- The health care delivery system will be stronger when the hospital and physician payments are not negotiated against each other, so a common contracting entity will be developed.

- Physician leadership and participation in all programs will be developed.

Organizational Performance and Capability The financial performance of the organization is another factor that drives the future options of the organization. The imperative is to seek capital and create capital reserves, not only for plant and equipment budgets, but also for payer settlement budgets and investment in the physician networks. The strategic directions for an organization with proper fund balances, reserves, or capital for necessary replenishment are very different from those of an organization without financial stability.

The payment mechanisms from Medicare and other major purchasers of care all reward least-cost resource use in health care delivery. These payment measures encourage the growth of postacute delivery services in subacute services and home care services. The organization, challenged to provide services across a spectrum of options, searches for least-cost options. The health care delivery system's ability to function efficiently, both clinically and financially, is essential for survival. Other factors important in maintaining a thriving market position are ensuring quality, measuring quality, and being competitive in technology and innovation in service delivery.

Selecting a category of quality indicators can help the organization to maintain market position. Quality indicator categories can include either those noted by credentialing agencies, such as the Joint Commission for the Accreditation of Healthcare Organizations or the National Committee for Quality Assurance (NCQA), or those factors noted in large databases with comparative performers, such as patient surveys, the Maryland project, or the Health Plan Employer Data and Information Set (HEDIS). The quality indicators used by the industry are most acceptable to other providers and payers. As the organization changes, new quality issues will have to be met concerning specific service goals or customer needs in specific markets. An organization ready to plan its future is prepared to evaluate and optimize operational efficiency, the provision of quality and value in service delivery, and technology and innovation.

A comparison of operating performance with industry standards and projected future requirements will help in setting goals to enhance productivity. With the onset of standardization in health care delivery, including outpatient care delivery and inpatient and support patient pathways, operational efficiency is required to perform in a manner that will attract and keep contracts.

The standardization of health care delivery provides the opportunity both to improve outcomes and to have a common high quality mode of practice. The use of clinical guidelines (for instance, practice guidelines to critical care pathways and care methodologies) is a means of ensuring quality under conditions of required deviation from care protocols. Guidelines are intended for the following purposes:

- helping physicians increase their efficiency
- improving decision making
- reducing costly variations in practice
- eliminating inappropriate procedures
- rationalizing approaches to care

The widespread use of guidelines may help reduce health care costs, and some commentators have forecast protection from malpractice suits.[II] Table 2-1 shows that while, overall, internists agree that guidelines are useful and will improve health care quality, there are some drawbacks to trying to apply them rigidly.

The improved operating efficiency occurs when services are streamlined and coordinated. Fee-for-service systems, without a primary care provider responsible for all service approval, do not reinforce coordination of care. Capitated care, with a primary care provider responsible for all service approval and global payment, reinforces the coordination for a patient among different services. There are benefits to services operating on common information or billing systems. Providers that have separate infrastructures may spend more time working out the coordination

TABLE 2-1. How Internists See Clinical Outcomes

Clinical Guidelines Are . . .	Percentage of Respondents Who "Agree" or "Strongly Agree"
Likely to be used in quality assurance	81%
Intended to improve quality of care	70%
Likely to be used in physician discipline	68%
A convenient source of advice	67%
Likely to improve quality of care	65%
Good educational tools	64%
Intended to decrease health care costs	61%
Likely to decrease physician reimbursement	38%
Likely to decrease physician satisfaction	34%
Unbiased synthesis of expert opinion	31%
Oversimplified or "cookbook opinion"	25%
Too rigid to apply to individual patients	24%
Likely to decrease health care costs	22%
A challenge to physician autonomy	21%
Likely to decrease malpractice suits	18%
Likely to decrease defensive practices	13%

Source: Adapted from *Annals of Internal Medicine* (June 1994).

aspects. The areas for enhanced coordination range from office-based medicine and acute care to subacute care and home care service delivery. Benchmarks and comparative database information improve operating efficiency, which strengthens the payer and purchaser positions.

Quality and proven value in service delivery are measured by technical capability, information, and customer services. NCQA is the accrediting agency for health plans. The NCQA standard includes 8 consumer satisfaction measures and 28 other criteria such as physician turnover, use of health care resources, and use rates per 1,000 members for selected medical care services. Market factors such as member disenrollment rates and premium costs have also been reported.[12] Many health plans, viewing themselves and their providers as overall systems, contractually mandate providers to comply with NCQA requirements.

With innovative and creative uses of equipment and procedures, it is essential to ensure the proper application of technology and service delivery. A greater emphasis on office practices, office-based procedures, ambulatory surgery, and postcare recovery centers underscores the shift away from acute care to office-based care. In addition, the shift now moves to more home care management, subacute care services, and other substitutes for the hospital-based expense in health care. However, organizations face the continuing challenge of ensuring proper environments and equipment to enable the hospital to offer acute care.

The organization's acceptance of change is partly a result of education and partly due to the compelling need for change. Benchmarking is used to educate and to determine what could be done as an effective means of change and goal setting. One director of hospital relations has said about benchmarking, "It's sort of structured learning. You always have to be on the lookout for someone who's doing something better than you."[13]

Current and Potential Financial Capability The financial capability of an organization has to provide sufficient funds to respond to its strategic directions. The primary requirement is to be able to transfer costs as payers continue to affect the shift in care. In addition, the ability to provide clinically appropriate care substitutes or innovative types of delivery to achieve the same outcome is both a clinical priority and a payment priority. The successful health care organization will be cost efficient, while maintaining updated resources. Richard Schrock, chief financial officer at Ohio State University Hospital, put it this way: "We keep looking at how we redefine resources. . . . That's the big issue when you talk about re-engineering. How do you shift from inpatient services to outpatient service, or a combination of that, and how do you get the right people in the right place?"[14]

The ability to manage both patients and resources resides in having the best information technology to show the resource use and utilization of the service delivery system. Again, this is a costly proposition. Many organizations see the hospital or the integrated system organization assuming the lead in developing this capability.

After a lengthy assessment of the organization's financial and clinical position, tactics may look like the following:

- Develop the best value position for managed care contracting.
- Respond to rapid technology development.
- Respond to changing delivery modalities with a full range of low-cost, best-value services.
- Either increase use of excess services or convert to other value-added, revenue-enhancing services.
- Provide supports to medical staff to respond to new pressures on physicians.
- Raise the operating margins and plan for an aging asset base.

Merger and Alliance Position   If being prepared calls for planning for relationship management, it also calls for collaboration planning. As in the various options of financial planning, the type of relationship and desired outcome drives the type of collaboration. In chapter 5, mechanisms and models for planning for collaborations are reviewed. Although strategic plans have to include a response to consumer needs, clinical practice efficacy, and financial viability, the means of accomplishing these responses in a financially constrained environment may call for collaborating with a range of partners, in a variety of ways.

Planning for networks and community care programs is essentially planning for collaboration. Such a direction comes from an initial analysis of the marketplace and the hospital. Just as there are financing options for different needs, there also are collaboration options for different purposes. Just as innovative systems can be creatively developed to achieve some ends, the development of coordinated care (through alliances, affiliations, networks, and cooperatives) can follow a variety of models. Potential collaborative providers will also be pursuing alliances in order to

- improve cost efficiency
- enhance one or more core competencies
- improve access to payer contracts
- improve access to a market area
- improve access to a primary care network
- obtain access to capital

By the time that this stage is considered, the opportunities for securing payer contracts, establishing a physician network, and assessing organizational directions and financial resources have become clear. As a result, there may be economic imperatives that facilitate a merger position. In addition to resource needs and mission, vision and values drive the organizational merger. In any case, there would be concrete reasons for considering some collaboration, whether it is a formal or informal corporate linkage. These organizational needs would become part of the consideration of the alliance needs as the flexible search for a partner, buyer, or ally commenced. There are also opportunities to form alliances with community service agencies and to establish links with the community by providing a variety of nonacute medical services.

The alliance position is more frequently considered than completed. Each health care provider organization has to consider what affiliation priorities they have and circumstances under which affiliations would make sense.

Getting and Keeping Customers As consolidation continues in the marketplace, there are new aspects to the supportive activities that get and keep groups of customers. The customers reached through payer contracts or employers are one group. The groups of customers reached through Medicare and Medicaid, whether those programs operate with a managed care component or not, may require special adjunct services to manage their care. In addition, the commitment to community health may require participation and outreach into new cultural groups in the service area, creating a new service delivery access. In this way, collaboration with other types of services, especially community groups and social service agencies, may take on new importance as a means of reaching out to special needs groups.

The traditional route to an acute care facility through the payer-physician relationship is deepened by the greater strategic emphasis of payer position and physician networks. The focus now becomes demonstrating value in each stage of the new organization's delivery system while dealing with the massive amount of change and renaming that is taking place during this transition.

Changing markets, changing customers, changing competitors, changing suppliers, changing distributors, and changing technology will lead to faster-paced market development. Life cycles of products and services will be shortened; repositioning in new service offerings and promotions raises marketing costs. The best means of responding to a rapidly changing marketplace is to remain current about the key changes and drivers of service selection and positioning. The characteristics of a successful market-driven organization are quality, service, speed, and adaptability.

To gain and keep customers, players must keep up with changes in distribution channels. They must use market research effectively, seeing how customer satisfaction affects provider selection and retention. The healthy community agenda has reshaped health care delivery and services, and players must meet these new demands.

Industry trends indicate that in the future the relationship between providers and members may come to resemble the retail industry, if employers step out of the preselection role. The experience in Minnesota illustrates these changes. "Most markets are in a stage of cost control, price wars and massive, sometimes anti-competitive consolidation," wrote one spectator. "Three health plans enroll most Minnesota residents and three major health systems own most Twin Cities hospitals. The Buyers Health Care Action Group, made up of 24 large employers, decided it wanted more competition. . . . HealthPartners coordinated a farmers' market where employees are given a premium allowance to spend as they choose at any of 14 contracted systems. Ultimately, employers determine the market. . . . Whatever buyers decide to reward, the health care system will create."[15]

If the distribution channels are likely to change, then the provider and payer strategies in providing value to the customer groups will correspondingly merge. The customer groups shift as public and private programs change their distribution channel. Public programs, operating on a prepaid basis, now move to a retail sales method and require the same direct marketing activities as retail sales. Although in this scenario employers still are purchasing health care coverage for their own employees, industry expert Jeff Goldsmith notes that the day may come when the selection process is turned over directly to the employee and family, and the issuance of vouchers will engender a system even closer to the retail model.[16]

Payers want to attract and retain their enrollees. Enrollee satisfaction is a value driver for payers, for employers, and even for the public programs. Research about the current expectations and anticipated preferences of the buyers—whether they are government payers, private payers, employers, or the direct customers themselves—sets the pace for the best results-oriented tactics. Under the fee-for-service model, every point of entry for a consumer should be defined. Under capitation, there are different criteria for selecting a network than in a fee-for-service system. It takes some time for an organization to become as effectively repositioned under capitation as in a fee-for-service system.

The consumer criteria for all services has to be identified and satisfied because choice defines the provider selection. The services must be up to the consumer's standard, and the specialty services must be up to the primary care provider's standards. The change requires primary care providers to refer to specialists in the medical community, which may require a strengthening of the specialty services. Capitation requires a medical community willing to work as a team to care for a designated patient population.

The most effective customer attraction and retention tactics have to be identified and developed. For an area with a shortage of primary care physicians where residents prefer local medical care, the opportunity to capture market share will be in establishing qualified primary care physicians with patient capacity. In a marketplace of young families, the premium and the maternity services may dominate the network selection. In a marketplace where there is uncertainty about employment, premium costs and copays may be more important that provider access.

Customer satisfaction drives the shape of the activities that form an organization. Despite what an organization eventually looks like or what network it may or may not be connected to, measuring satisfaction is a hallmark of successful organizations that rejuvenate themselves even while they are evolving.

A customer's selection of health care providers in a fee-for-service, relatively unmanaged, marketplace is more complex than in a marketplace with more managed care. In a marketplace with less managed care, depending on the insurance provisions, the interest in and affiliation with a primary care physician may be less frequent than in a marketplace with a payer-required primary care physician. Also, the selection of specialists may be more important than when customers are required to use a specific medical community. Therefore, depending on the marketplace, the progress of the managed care penetration and the health service habits and preferences are drivers of what customers expect and will seek.

In any marketplace, market assessments and market research need to be current on the following issues:

- customer perception and willingness to use services
- customer habits in selection and use of health services
- customer willingness to switch and reasons for switching health services or payers
- customer perception of change in services, corporate structure, or affiliation

With consolidation in health care, determining a customer's perspective on the levels of change is necessary to continue to promote the value of the organization and define the actual benefits of the changes.

Market research is useful to confirm that the network development direction has some level of value to the consumer, to confirm how customers view the health care organization, to measure the impact of other area providers, and to test the appeal of value-added factors that the organization may currently or potentially offer to gain new users, affiliated households, or covered lives.

Health plans and providers alike are scrambling to raise customer satisfaction. The keys to customer retention are obtaining high satisfaction ratings and giving as few reasons for switching providers as possible. Providers are measuring their patients' satisfaction in terms of their own providers and against industry figures. Providers are interested in patient

satisfaction systems that provide access to large databases of patient satisfaction measurements. Satisfaction measures have evolved from testing
patient satisfaction with "hotel" services (for example, food, parking, and
room quality) to testing encounters and outcomes.

The NCQA requires measures of patient satisfaction as part of the
commitment to health care quality. At the same time, because of the
importance of the primary care physician, most of the surveys following
the NCQA standards also measure satisfaction with access, communication outcomes, and satisfaction with both doctor and practice.

Customer satisfaction includes the satisfaction with and access to
specialists. The results may require shoring up specialty and ancillary services. A network has to include specialists who are acceptable to primary
care providers. This relationship flows both ways. Specialists should have
confidence in the primary care providers' clinical capabilities. In an area
with many health care providers, primary care providers who are referring to specialists in other medical communities (at other providers) are
not participating in a unified medical community. Involving them in the
refinement of services for which there are non-network referrals (such as
oncology, pulmonary disease care, or cardiology) will more likely inten-
sify their commitment to referring locally.

In a fee-for-service market that is becoming a managed care market,
factors such as service awareness, service use satisfaction, and dissatis-
faction ratings are important in determining future use. In a fee-for-
service market moving toward capitation or increased managed care, the
affiliation with the primary care providers and the willingness to switch
to one's primary care providers are important to measure, as well as perceptions and willingness to use key services that are part of the health
care system selection factors (such as maternity services or emergency
services).

Whether because of anticipated legislation or because of a voluntary
shift in direction, the new emphasis on healthy communities represents
a significant change in how providers viewed health care needs in the
early 1990s. A healthy community is not a social concept. It is intended
to accomplish the following:

- demonstrate value to payers and employers in response to broad-
  based concerns over health care costs
- respond to the proposals for health reform, including the prepaid
  government contracts (Medicare/Medicaid)
- inventory community health needs and respond appropriately
- develop more outreach and intervention in high-risk populations

The increased attention to capitation, both as a means of payment
and a modality for delivering care, heightened the clear need to make
long-term contract with those enrollees whose health care is now the

purview of the provider. Perhaps that is because the preparation for capitation means an investment in those who are part of the health care
delivery system. Perhaps social responsibility flared up in the face of
drastically cut services and brought about the increased attention to providing care for communities.

As a strategic initiative, quality has become essential in measuring
both processes and outcomes. Healthy practices, healthy outcomes, and
preventive practices have become important. Employers looking for
demonstrated value and payers seeking to reward quality providers coin-
cide with providers instilling healthy practices both in communities and
across provider networks.

Step 7. Develop an Action Plan

The identified strategy conclusions must be put into actionable statements. Actionable items may be somewhat fluid (though not necessarily
linear) and customizable as implementation progresses. Because those
responsible for the actions may not be directly involved with planning, it
is critical to develop a strategy to instill in employees the vision, mission,
and strategy.

Sources for Actions to Be Taken There are many sources of information to help determine what actions need to be taken. These include
a data review in response to the external factors, market research of the
needs of the current health care delivery organization's users and area
residents, and a technical review of capability.

Expected Outcomes of Actions Taken The expected outcomes
would include the following six items, based on the strategic planning
processes:

1. compiling a vision statement
2. preparing a values statement
3. articulating positions decisions
   - payer position
   - physician network position
   - organizational position
   - financial position
   - community position
   - alliance position
4. listing action items in each category
5. profiling the future organization
6. teaming goals of financial and clinical volume with an overall
   view of where the organization is headed

Suppose the organization seeks an affiliation with another organization. Key criteria that make an affiliation problematic might be leadership, control over the financial resources, and access to capital. The establishment of thresholds helps to preset the terms under which the initiative should be considered. This step may be saved for the major initiatives, such as those affecting the organization on a corporate level. For business-specific and approach-specific initiatives project managers might set their own thresholds, subject to approval of senior management and reported through to the planning committee. Local criteria would be in line with the established benchmarks for operation.

PAST PROBLEMS WITH STRATEGIC PLAN DEVELOPMENT

Strategic plan development has been through several generations of improvements, often based on failures of the past. Overreliance on facts is often a path toward faulty forecasts. Supreme faith in a plan that excludes the participation of key stakeholders can also be detrimental. Strategies establish incentives for staff and create greater flexibility to allow for new external factors and operational creativity. Participation and inclusion are important here; however, vision drives the process to position an organization in a changing environment.

Strategy, in and out of health care, is frequently redefined, indicating a high level of interest in a discipline that is still being revised as a result of its many apparent failures. (See chapter 4 for a discussion of the problems with strategic plan implementation.) The problems point to the need for greater unity in a workforce, more emphasis on organizational culture change, and the pressing need for leadership.

For the past several decades, business literature has continually reinvented strategy applications, strategic success, and elements for making insightful conclusions that map the road to change. The failures of strategy, however, are attributable to many factors, including

- lack of commitment
- lack of employee alignment
- cumbersome processes
- inflexible planning systems

Lack of Commitment

A service delivery system cannot be successful without the complete commitment of its workers. Employees need technical competence and imagination to look for new ways to respond to key needs. The organizational vision and values guide the allocation of resources and are reflected in the way in which patients, employees, and other customer groups are treated. A number of factors lead to lack of commitment, including

- *Lack of information:* Employees who are unaware of either the directions of the organization or the driving factors behind the direction have no reason or context to understand the strategic direction. For plans developed by a small group that are not shared with employees and not discussed with the senior or middle management, employees have no ability to make a commitment to the decentralized implementation. Affiliated physicians who are not apprised of or consulted about the organization's future are likely to feel alienated from the strategic future.
- *Lack of a shared vision:* Alliances require a shared vision that, if missing, leads to a lack of commitment. Management issues and conflicts arise, and when a common framework is missing, these minor tremors can lead to major earthquakes.
- *Lack of shared incentives:* For employees and affiliated physicians, the lack of shared incentives for success, on both a personal and divisional basis, also contributes to the lack of commitment to an organization's future. Performance management systems that reward individual performance without being tied to the organizational success will fail to get commitment needed for strategic change. Linking financial to organizational success creates one kind of incentive system.
- *Lack of leadership investment in the planning process:* Strategic plan development works only if management is committed to support its development. The lack of investment in the planning process by senior management, from the head of the organization on, jeopardizes employee ownership and inhibits successful strategic plan development. Without leadership to present, validate, and reinforce the vision and values in management actions, there is no unity in pursuing the strategic future. Managers may become sidetracked by solving immediate operational problems outside the long-term strategic plan. Such short-term fixes may sidetrack or derail the long-term plan, in both implementation and the way resources are spent. Figure 2-2 is a checklist of the top 10 warning signs that something is wrong with strategic planning.

Lack of Employee Alignment

Another challenge for the planning process is having the right participants and establishing a milieu for others to become in engaged in implementation. The participants include those who directly implement the new

FIGURE 2-2. Top 10 Warning Signs That Something Is Wrong with the Strategic Plan

1. Top management assumes that it can delegate the planning function to an outside planner.
2. Top management becomes so engrossed in current problems that it spends insufficient time on long-range planning, and the process becomes discredited among other managers and staff.
3. Company goals are not suitable as a basis for formulating long-range plans.
4. Front-line personnel are not involved in the planning process.
5. Plans are not used as standards for measuring managerial performance.
6. The climate in the company is resistant to planning.
7. Comprehensive planning is separated from the entire management process.
8. The system is so formal that it lacks flexibility, looseness, and simplicity and restrains creativity.
9. Top management does not review with departmental and divisional heads the long-range plans that they have developed.
10. Top management consistently rejects the formal planning mechanism by making intuitive decisions.

Adapted from Henry Mintzberg, *The Rise and Fall of Strategic Planning.* (New York: The Free Press, 1994), pp. 174–75.

directions and those who have to provide the necessary infrastructure. The right milieu includes both the climate to favor strategy implementation and the process for departments and divisions to have some flexibility in the implementation. This flexibility allows them to translate their values and vision into actions, for which they must then be held accountable, measured, and rewarded. To meet both the company vision and local marketplace realities, the plan must allow some freedom for divisional plans.

Aligning employees involves communicating the vision, helping them see their role in its attainment, and acquiring the proper talent to engage in the new functions and activities of the organization. This activity will help employees invest in the future of the organization. The use of teams as a means of facilitating strategic initiatives will allow input at the operational level that is necessary for successful strategic planning.

The organizational loyalty of employees has changed in the last several decades. The means of obtaining employee commitment requires more creativity than in the past. Managers look to encourage commitment and buy-in rather than imposing rule and expecting blind loyalty. Henry Mintzberg has written, "The more clearly the strategy is articulated, the more deeply embedded it becomes, in both the habits of the organization and the minds of its people."[17]

When allocating resources for projects, there may be a temptation to consider who is sponsoring them rather than their pure value to the organization. Such favoritism lacks vision about where the organization is going and shows deficient decision making. If a planning process relies on decision making that is based on those who scream the loudest or who have the biggest offices, it could fail because of a lack of support. The details of strategy articulation and its implementation as a means of gaining employee alignment are discussed more fully in chapter 4.

Cumbersome Processes

Mistakes are made in planning because of poor process management, a lack of clarity about financial resources, a lack of analytic data to support directions, or a lack of imagination to support strategic planning. Inflexible plans dictate the direction of the organization, but they neither account for existent processes and capabilities, allow opportunity to shape initiatives, nor allow the operational staff to achieve optimal outcomes.

The decision-making style of a management team that relies on last-minute decisions based on intuition fails to take advantage of timely factual assessment. In contrast, an organization can process so much information that decisions are not made; the process becomes cumbersome and an end in itself. Strategy failures are partly due to focusing too much on information and too little on results. The seduction of "analysis paralysis" is that endless meetings and consensus building make it seem that work is being done, but in focusing on the process, a window of opportunity may be missed.

The goal is for all participants to realize their professional interests in a visionary, practical, professionally appropriate end-product plan. Recognizing that each constituency may bring different values to the table, the process would start with open discussion about shared values, then move to the formulation of a common vision and the implementation of a strategy to carry out the vision. Although analytical evaluation and thoughtfully interpreted consensus are important tools to direct an organization, it is important to understand the players and the agendas they bring to the process. The values for the organization, both in the way business was conducted in the past and will be conducted in the future, are useful in articulating the means for achieving the results. The values dictate how the result is achieved, in a fashion consistent with the way management wishes to do business. Clarification also aids in the planning process, as does an agreement by participants to take ownership of the planning results.

Inflexible Planning Process

The strategic plan can be perfect on paper, but if it does not have practical application, it is an academic exercise, not a plan. Peter Drucker has noted that few businesses raise the key questions for strategy related to the actual task and expected outcomes. He writes of a company where

> a planning staff of 45 brilliant people carefully prepared "strategic scenarios" down to minute details. It was first-class work and stimulating reading, everybody admitted. But it had minimum operational impact. A new CEO asked, "What is the task?" His answer: "It isn't to predict the future. It is to give our businesses directions and goals and the strategy to attain these goals." It took four years of hard work and several false starts. But now the planning people—still about the same number—work through only three questions for each of the company's businesses: What market standing does it need to maintain leadership? What innovative performance does it need to support the needed market standing? What rate of return is the minimum needed to earn the cost of capital?[18]

CONCLUSION

Strategic plan development has four essential components: (1) a consensus as to the challenges and opportunities facing the organization; (2) a vision of what the organization is becoming; (3) sufficient analytical information to contextualize the organization's performance in the marketplace; and (4) a platform of strategic directions. By following the seven steps of strategic plan development, the organization can identify its strengths and weaknesses and resolve short- and long-term challenges.

References

1. Whit Spaulding, *A Deer in the Lobby: An Irreverent Look at American Management* (Birmingham, Mich.: Barn Press, 1991).

2. James Moore, "The Death of Competition," *Fortune* (Apr. 15, 1996): p. 143.

3. Burt Nanus, *Visionary Leadership* (San Francisco: Jossey-Bass, 1992), p. 34.

4. Adapted from Leadership Studies International, Value Audit Workshop (Oct. 11, 1991).

5. Leonard D. Goodstein, Timothy M. Nolan, and William J. Pfeiffer, *Applied Strategic Planning* (San Diego: Pfeiffer & Co., 1992), p. 146.

6. C. K. Prahalad, Liam Faley, and Robert M. Randall, "A Strategy for Growth: The Role of Core Competencies in the Corporation," in *The Portable MBA in Strategy,* by Liam Faley and Robert M. Randall (New York: Wiley, 1994), p. 258.

7. Henry Mintzberg, *The Rise and Fall of Strategic Planning* (New York: The Free Press, 1994), pp. 209–10.

8. David Burda, "FTC Approves Two Way Merger in Maine," *Modern Healthcare* (Mar. 20, 1995): 17.

9. Mintzberg, *Strategic Planning,* pp. 337–40.

10. *Healthcare PR & Marketing News* (Oct. 31, 1996): 3.

11. Rhonda Bergman, "Getting the Goods on Guidelines," *Hospitals and Health Networks* (Oct. 10, 1994): 70–74.

12. *Renaissance for Health Care: Environmental Assessment 1995/1996* (Chicago: American Hospital Association), p. 49.

13. Rhonda Bergman, "Hitting the Mark," *Hospitals and Health Networks* (Apr. 20, 1994): 48–50.

14. William O. Cleverley, *1996 Investment Management Institute Guide to Managing Financial Assets for Healthcare Systems, Hospitals, HMOs and Large Clinics* (Greenwich, Conn.: IMI), pp. 15-17.

15. *Modern Healthcare* (Sept. 5, 1996): p. 88. This story was based on the remarks of George Halvorson.

16. Jeff Goldsmith, speech given to the Society for Healthcare Strategy and Market Development, Atlanta (Sept. 30, 1996).

17. Mintzberg, *Strategic Planning,* p. 72.

18. Peter Drucker, *Managing for the Future: The 1990s and Beyond* (New York: Dutton, 1992), p. 100.

3

Assessment of the Environment

The true measure of any society is not what it knows but what it does with what it knows.

—*Warren Bennis*

Executive Summary

Strategic plan development requires an assessment of the external environment to see how industry drivers for change can be applied to health care. The ability to review relevant data for an environmental analysis requires consideration of national trends for business generally and health care specifically. A variety of models are available that can be applied to action planning, each of which shape health care in terms of any organization's ability to proceed, perform, or respond. These factors also help to identify potential scenarios for the health organization's future vision.

INTRODUCTION

During the past two decades, the health care industry has evolved into an integrated system of care. Many of the stand-alone hospitals and independent physicians have been replaced by systems that are now fully integrated—both in terms of service delivery and financing.

The health care industry now comprises a variety of types of providers and services. Some organizations provide a full range of services, from inpatient acute care to specialty services provided at satellite locations. Other health care organizations have crossed into the financing area, forming their own HMOs and preferred provider organizations (PPOs) and hiring their own contract physicians. Still others have developed into niche players, focusing on specialty services and carving out a narrow range of services.

This chapter reviews the framework for gathering information for strategic plan development and updates, beginning with a scan of industry drivers for strategic change and their relevance to health care. It also looks at the provider-payer landscape. In addition, the chapter discusses several models and methods for industry analysis. Finally, the chapter reviews collaborative partner selection and discusses lessons learned about performing environmental assessments.

IDENTIFYING INDUSTRY DRIVERS

Industry drivers are those key elements that change the payment systems or the supply and demand for health care services. Thus the first step in an industry analysis is to develop the list of industry drivers. These are derived from national health care payer reports, national provider commentaries, and regional industry analyses. From these, inferences are drawn about how the industry will change, how the market will respond in three to five years, and what the organization might start to look like during that time.

Industry drivers affect the environment and the makeup of the core business of an organization. The economy is one example of an industry driver; a fruitful economy will promote buying and spending. Customer base is also an essential driver of any industry; identifying the customer groups and meeting their various needs for any product or service drives the success of any organization. Another important industry driver is human resources. Whether employees are the vital connection to customers in a service industry or the determinants of quality in production, the most important resource of a company is its staff. Employees are also responsible for delivering clinical services and using available diagnostic and treatment technologies—other drivers that often form the core of the health care organization.

The extent to which the industry operates within regulatory parameters greatly affects its business opportunities and situation. The presence of regulations has implications for strategic decision making, as well as for payment or reimbursement mechanisms. In the health care industry, for example, payment is usually made by insurance companies or government programs (rather than by the actual user), and usually from multiple buyers (for instance, the payer and the employer). As a result, it is important to distinguish between the payers and the consumers (patients). Postindustrial businesses focus on the customer, where the buyer is different from the actual user, suggesting that both demographic issues and payer perspectives are a requisite focus of any postindustrial strategic assessment.

Because each of these drivers—economics; demographics; human resources; clinical treatment, clinical practice guidelines, and technology;

regulatory and political activities; and finance and payment mechanisms—profoundly affects the health care industry, they will be discussed in detail in the following subsections.

Economics

Trends in the national economy greatly affect the overall environment in which the health care delivery industry operates. Inflation, interest rates, productivity, corporate profit margins, and employment indicators are relevant to potential growth and change in health care delivery. The national economic position often generates changes in government spending. These changes affect the Health Care Financing Administration (HCFA), which funds Medicare, the largest purchaser of health care coverage for those 65 years of age and older. The health care delivery system often models clinical service delivery around this most user-intensive payer—in this case the elderly, who use two to three times the amount of health care services as the nonelderly.

The overall condition of the economy also influences employers' decisions to offer and fund health coverage for their employees. Economic factors cited as drivers of movements to halt health care spending and fund health care delivery in a wholly different way (at least starting with the proposed national health reform proposals this decade) include

- growing annual costs of providing health insurance for a typical employee
- increased health care spending at a national level, as a percentage of the gross national product (GNP)
- growth rates of medical expenditures leading to private and public purchasers of services, and the subsequent initiatives at the state level to manage spending by health care facilities and payers

Demographics

Changes in the demographics of a region and the nation affect health care delivery and certainly the focus of those served. Two easily identifiable demographic groups are the elderly and the baby-boomer generation. The conjunction of these two with the aging of the baby-boomers will obviously have a substantial, but still evolving, impact on the industry.

National demographic changes are indicators of where resources will be spent in shaping and responding to health care needs and developing services. Regional demographic movements point to resource needs and opportunities to enhance community health. Local demographic differences show changing claims on the health care system and needs that can be addressed immediately to avoid potential problems. Population trends are monitored to identify opportunities in allocating health care resources. From policy comes program development, from which support and reimbursement trends are set.

Changes in population trends affect the health care delivery system. Economic fluctuations influence the dependence on public programs for those with limited incomes. The growth of the elderly population and changes in lifestyles have an effect on the present and future Medicare programs. An increase in the rate of homeless people—caused by unemployment, de-institutionalization of the mentally ill, substance abuse, and lack of affordable housing—has contributed to a corresponding increase in poverty levels.[1]

In addition, the presence of diverse ethnic groups who may not be reached by the current delivery system requires different configurations to ensure access. Indicators of cultural diversity among the customer population are important triggers to health care delivery organizations to offer services in the languages and traditions of their diverse customer groups. National policy makers also rely on demographic data to identify and deal with health care issues concerning illegal immigrants. Therefore, the use of demographic information—updated as frequently as possible—is not only a good planning tool, but an important aspect of developing a competent culture.

Human Resources

Partly because of the last decade of increased spending, and partly because of the labor-intensive nature of this industry, the role of human resources is an essential strategic element in health care delivery. Laura Avakian, senior vice president of CareGroup and Beth Israel Deaconess Medical Center (formerly Beth Israel Hospital) underscores the importance of employees: "Bright aggressive human resources people have to move forward in the language of business, the discussion of how to capitalize on human beings' contributions. We need everyone to be highly energized about delivering goals."[2]

Changes in clinical service practices and payer requirements have brought massive changes to health care practice. The demand for key staff roles has created market shortages and surpluses. The pressure to reduce health care delivery costs means that there will be a continuing call for training, as well as a continuing call for cross-training among many roles and duties. The broader range of health care delivery options has been accompanied by a change in clinical care settings. What has been provided in the acute care hospital setting may now be moved to home care, outpatient care, or subacute care, while acute care services are "downsized" and staff shift jobs. The increasing importance of allied health professionals has created more demand for such professionals. The physician maldistribution across specialties and geographic areas has continued to plague many health care delivery organizations.

Just as there is more diversity among patients, so too there is more diversity among health care employees. Greater adaptation to the needs and requirements of both cultural differences and family issues among its staff has forced the health care industry to address issues relating to child care, family care, and other specialty benefit programs.

Clinical Treatment, Clinical Practice Guidelines, and Technology

Changes both in the diagnosis and treatment of disease and injuries have helped basic sciences develop new sets of capabilities.

Clinical Treatment If the 1980s brought advances in diagnosis and minimally invasive surgery, then the 1990s and beyond will bring more capabilities in biotechnology. In addition, there will be an enhanced capability in predicting disease based on a person's genetic makeup. Biotechnology is enhancing the predictive capacity to understand disease based on genetic makeup and to manage an illness before symptoms emerge.

Another clinical change is immunotherapy, which stimulates the immune system to heal wounds and help with the growth and repair of organs and tissues. The implication in medical care is the expanded ability to care for diseases before they fully emerge. With enhanced ability to recognize and treat diseases comes the identification of other diseases. Certainly, the identification of AIDS and other communicable diseases has increased pressures on health care providers to manage infectious diseases. With these advancements, the attention to public health becomes essential. In some situations, prevention and education become relevant in forestalling diseases, rather than merely treating them once they occur.

Clinical Practice Guidelines Clinical practice guidelines, used to avoid error through standardizing care and to enhance quality, introduce a new technical competence factor into health care delivery. The anticipated onset of capitation as a dominant payment mechanism also has introduced the concept of standardized care. This is a new approach to clinical practice, as is the search for least expensive care in a variety of settings. Practice guidelines thus help to reduce the variations and possibility of error among health care organizations faced with new directives to cut costs and standardize care.

Technology Another recent advancement is the availability of information technology. Automation has enhanced reporting capabilities, enabled instant retrieval of patient records, and offered computer-generated reminders with practice guideline options. The use of telemedicine for education, consultation, and treatment is especially important in the delivery of medical care in rural areas or areas with a scarcity of resources. As patient care settings have become more diverse, monitoring and compatible care guidelines will be needed.

Regulatory and Political Activities

Health care is and has been a highly regulated industry. Public funding since World War II helped to build large numbers of acute care facilities, and resultant regulatory activities have spawned the modern health care industry. The public payers—Medicare and Medicaid—lead the trends in health care payments. The prepaid managed care system used in both public programs became the model for many proposed versions of national health reform. When free market dictates took over, the public payers focused on paying for health care on a "disinflationary" basis. Public programs and employers want lower costs, and payers—both public and private—are forced to respond. Consumers' demands for choice have impeded the anticipated advantages from forming networks and engaging large contracts. Health care providers now have to differentiate based on actual and perceived levels of indicators, including quality indicators, avoidable error rates, and costs.

The push for disinflationary costs means that there will be fewer funds available for the health care delivery system. The challenge to do more with less has brought a series of operational management challenges, the renewed attention to cost management, and a focus on least cost/high quality care.

Regulatory issues faced in health care include the extent to which the federal government delegates power to the states. The traditional tax-exempt status and other benefits of health care organizations will continue to be under scrutiny. Likewise, increased scrutiny related to antitrust concerns affect the formation of mergers and networks.

Finance and Payment Mechanisms

The way that health care providers offer their services and receive payments has changed. Declining reimbursement payments pressure providers to decrease costs yet develop payment terms that balance financial requirements with the cost of clinical service.

The pressure in this decade to decrease costs, resulting in slower rates of cost increases, has been appreciated by the buyers. Lower rate increases and a choice of providers are the criteria for employer and customer selection. Those payers that provide greater provider choices are preferred. That enrollment in PPOs is outpacing that of HMOs underscores the importance—both to employers and employees—of the preference for choice of provider. Jeff Goldsmith has presented a strong message rejecting the limitation of choice of the provider. He comments that the failure of national health reform meant that government restriction of provider choice, even to achieve cost decreases, was ultimately unacceptable to the marketplace.[3]

The private health insurance market, offering a range of options in managed care, as well as being the sole product offered by HMOs and PPOs, is diversifying. Kaiser's creation of multiple products and contracts with providers in selected markets is an indicator that too-narrow health plans have failed to succeed in the marketplace. Capitated payments have meant a shift of economic risk for over- or underutilization of services from the payers to the providers. Even the use of diagnosis-related group (DRG)-based payment initiated by the HCFA shifted utilization incentives from payers to providers. Actuarial methodologies to examine actual cost and utilization behavior are now being used by providers as well as payers.

The perceived advantages of direct contracting, and the growth of public sector managed care, require constant redefinition of both the costs and the modalities of care. The changes in Medicare, often the bulk of physicians' and hospitals' businesses, incorporate both capital expense reimbursement and physician payment reform.

THE PAYER/PROVIDER LANDSCAPE

Understanding the industry drivers provides one piece of the industry analysis. Another is fleshing out the organization's view of other payers and providers in the marketplace.

Other Payers

In addition to its relationship with its current payers, an organization must assess other payers who are active in the marketplace, or have the potential to become active payers. This assessment is done by identifying the payers that are used by area employers and residents. Area employers and residents can be surveyed to determine prior payer preference, current payer use, attitudes toward payers, and reasons for enrolling with specific payers. Identifications of valued characteristics of each payer aid the positioning of the provider in future contract negotiations.

A variety of other factors are important with respect to payers. Market successes in enrollment, turnover, change in corporate accounts, commercial products, and Medicare/Medicaid participation provide some indicators of payer capability. Claims-made ratios provide another indicator of use. Understanding the financial solvency of the plan is also important to evaluate. The success of each plan in a marketplace is important in making conclusions and entering into negotiation.

Although the active payers in the local market may be easily identified, other payers could have the potential to enter the service area. A payer active in the secondary service area, for example, may be under pressure to expand its market share. An option might be to expand into the primary service area as a means of extending its own business. Failing to consider potential payers can leave significant gaps in understanding the industry.

Other Providers

A review of competing providers falls into two categories: those that directly affect the service area or life of the health care organization through overlapping interests; and those that do not directly affect the organization, but could serve as role models.

Providers That Directly Compete with the Organization Those providers that directly compete with the organization usually want to provide care for the same patients, target the same physicians, serve the same geographic locale, or contract for the same services with payers. These competitors, however, can be attractive candidates for alliance (discussed later in this chapter).

A review of comparable providers includes the following information:

- clinical service profile (a detailed list of all services available through a health care organization)
- clinical performance
- cost and charge position
- participating payers
- scope of medical staff (including the primary care provider's geographic location and practice mode, as well as a list of the specialists available)
- perception by area consumers of area providers

Benefits of looking at other providers: Most health care organizations may seem similar. Identifying key differences and then measuring them as seen by the end users—the payers and the area employers—for the level of value placed on those differences will lead to useful decision making. Although this provider assessment may appear to focus on similar organizations, the provider assessment is best done with the full range of health care-related services available in or to a geographic marketplace.

Looking at other providers in the marketplace is a practice that is useful for a variety of reasons, including the following:

- *sensitization,* which challenges an organization's existing assumptions about other organizations' capabilities
- *benchmarking,* which provides a set of specific measures comparing an organization with other providers
- *legitimization,* which justifies proposals and persuades members of an organization of the feasibility and desirability of a chosen course of action
- *inspiration,* which gives people new ideas on how to solve problems by identifying what other firms have done in similar circumstances
- *planning,* which uses competitor analysis to assist the formal planning process
- *decision making,* which contributes to creativity and range in operational and tactical decision making by line managers[4]

Information about other providers also is useful in identifying the best practices in terms of clinical efficiency, service capability, and cost. Studies of other organizations can also help to identify services that are missing in a full-service complement and to determine whether to include them. Although competitor analyses are recognized as primary to the planning process, support for decision making is also an essential reason to study other providers. Information about what other providers have done helps line managers make decisions about how to proceed in specific situations.

Benefits of competitor tracking: Regular competitor tracking is an important planning responsibility. When profiling providers, include an analysis of competitors' market shares, payer contracts, medical staff profiles, ratios of primary care providers to secondary care providers, and ratios of primary care providers to the service area population. It is important to evaluate financial capabilities, services provided, and newly offered and planned services. For example, a major provider in a secondary service area with decreased utilization may plan to downsize acute care services or establish satellite facilities in the primary service area to extend its own services and compete for market share. Knowing this in advance will help an organization plan and act strategically.

For example, one payer had contracts with loose terms with several similar providers in a service area. The payer announced an exclusive arrangement that directed the volume that had gone to several providers to now go to a single provider, without allowing for competition. The excluded providers reviewed the performance of the selected provider, and found that it had experienced a three-year trend of declining volume.

A competitor tracking program would have enabled the other providers in the marketplace to anticipate such a dramatic move. They could have potentially secured their own volume with different contract terms and not risked it on this payer.

Models for innovative service delivery that indicate how organizations can work together are extremely useful as a means of inspiring possibilities within a specific marketplace. For example, one newspaper report that "New York City has reached out even as far as northwestern Connecticut, going over state lines to establish an affiliation. The affiliation is a 'loose' alliance [that] will also potentially include shared purchasing and managed care contracting. Regional reach blurs with the outreach efforts of some health care organizations."[5]

Providers That Serve as Role Models Role model organizations are ones that appear to respond effectively to the industry drivers in their environment. Role models can be found in more mature organizations, such as experienced physician practice management firms; health care systems that have a greater percentage of managed care penetration in the marketplace; or payers that operate with a larger percentage of provider capitation contracts. The characteristics that make them able to respond effectively, as well as the innovations that make them unusual, are notable. More important are the driving pressures that cause them to respond.

Regional role models or leading edge institutions should also be assessed. Even organizations with past leadership records are worth tracking; their reactions to external threats and opportunities may provide insight for the future of other organizations.

MODELS FOR PERFORMING AN INDUSTRY ANALYSIS

Progress in the planning process requires self-evaluation in the context of the industry. A variety of models exist for conducting industry assessments. The most useful applications for the health care industry are SWOT analysis and competitive forces.

SWOT Analysis: Identifying Strengths, Weaknesses, Opportunities, and Threats

Identifying strengths, weaknesses, opportunities, and threats (SWOT) is an essential tool for an organization in the throes of strategic plan development. SWOT analysis strengthens action planning by matching results across categories (that is, identification of internal strengths can reveal outside opportunities, whereas knowledge of weaknesses can prepare an organization for external threats).

Implementing this analytic tool for strategic planning requires two steps:

1. Gather data on internal performance (for instance, level of efficiency) and external environment (for instance, identified marketplace needs). With this assessment a picture is developed about how the organization fits in the scope of current realities. It can be used to review data on the competitor organizations as well.
2. Review the organization's capability to become the one defined in the vision statement. The SWOT factors will play a role in determining what kinds of challenges the organization will face in achieving its vision.

The range of information collected about organizations and service is based both on intuition (organizational culture) and analytic facts (composition of medical staff in the provider network). The range of information has to be taken into consideration when looking at a strategic profile. A "soft" framework for profiling purposes poses the danger of using subjective data in the position estimation. Opinions about organizations are by nature subjective and will be at best inconclusive. A subjective assessment must have a specific analysis attached to it; it is a profile that can be developed by staff, and reviewed and added to by management. The final subjective and objective analysis will be ready for review and discussion by oversight groups or even a board committee. Table 3-1 lists qualitative and quantitative measures that need to be evaluated as a part of the SWOT analysis.

Whether something is a strength or weakness, or an opportunity or threat, depends on the position of the organization being analyzed, relative to its competitors. Once the lists of items are developed for these four categories, the internal factors should be compared with the external factors. The internal factors about an organization should be matched up to the external factors from the environmental assessment. Any item under any of the categories may have a strategic implication in and of itself, but it has a more compelling meaning when compared with the other factors. This is an essential part of a SWOT analysis.

Use the following scenarios and guidelines to lead the organization toward action steps in the planning process:

- *Organizational strengths match opportunities.* The organization has the internal strength to maximize external opportunity.
- *Internal strengths do not respond to external threats.* Caution: The organization's internal capability must be developed, possibly through affiliation, merger, or acquisition.

TABLE 3-1. SWOT Analysis Categories

Internal Strengths and Weaknesses	External Opportunities and Threats
Financial feasibility (profit or loss)	Industry analysis
Level of efficiency	Secondary consumer and area resident information
Level of flexibility to adjust to variable volume	Area and regional provider assessments
Inventory level	Consumer market research
Quality measures	Community needs assessment
Staff and physician satisfaction	Payer assessment and position
Level of internal communication	Service comparison
Level of coordination across services and departments	Future scenarios
Throughput efficiency	
Access for new users, customers, and patients	
Ability to implement innovation in services and products	
Current compared to past and potential change in total cycle time	
Comparative performance to external industry standards	
Staff and physician productivity and turnover (level of stability	
Fit with future scenarios	
Fit with the vision statement	

- *Internal organizational strengths do not match threats or opportunities.* Reassess: The strengths may relate to projected threats or opportunities, depending on the way the future is envisioned by the strategic planning team. If the strengths are relevant to the future or projected scenarios, then they should be protected and enhanced. If the strengths are not relevant to the current or foreseeable environment, then the organization should reconsider any investments in maintaining them and investigate whether those resources would be better spent elsewhere.
- *Internal organizational weaknesses do not match external threats or opportunities.* Assess: The weaknesses may be vulnerabilities for the projected environmental scenarios. If they are not relevant, then the extent to which they are real weaknesses should be examined.

- *Internal weaknesses do not match external opportunities.* Caution: Seeking an ally or developing a short-term fix may be needed to manage this opportunity.
- *Internal weaknesses do match external threats.* Caution: The internal capability is not present. Consider long-term measures: Develop other internal solutions to counter persistent threats.
- *External threats do not match internal strengths or weaknesses.* Consider development: Any threat to a service or organization in which the organization or service is neutral means that some distinctive capability should be developed, either directly or through a collaborative process.
- *External opportunities do not match internal strengths or weaknesses.* First, evaluate whether the organization even has the capability to respond to the opportunity, regardless of strengths and weaknesses. The organization can contract for the necessary provider to meet the opportunity, or develop the capability internally if time permits. Another means of responding to an opportunity is to collaborate with another organization that has more or complementary capabilities.
- *External threats do not match internal strengths or weaknesses.* Evaluate the practical impact of the threat on the organization in a very concrete fashion. If it still rates it as a threat, then reevaluate the organization's ability to respond to it. The organization may seek an affiliation to bring in greater talent or practical assets to respond appropriately. Assess whether other organizations are also threatened, and investigate alliances. Determine what an organization will be able to tolerate under all scenarios.

Framework for Assessing Competitor Forces

Michael Porter's 1980 book, *Competitive Strategy*, offers another framework for competitor assessment, using a long-standing model of forces that drive industry competition. This model assesses the following activities driving an industry:

- rivalry of area providers (with the assessment of competitors)
- threat of new providers (with the examination of potential entrants)
- threat of substitute products or services (with the assessment of substitutes)
- bargaining power of buyers (with the assessment of the buyers)
- bargaining power of suppliers (with the assessment of suppliers)[6]

New entrants, substitutes, and changes are affecting existing health care delivery organizations in most regional markets. For example, payers are now in the business of being providers. Home care services are replacing inpatient acute care services. Many existing acute care hospitals will close partly because of service delivery changes, lost volume because of payer contracts, or high costs. Some acute care hospitals that could not afford the necessary capital investment in their plants and equipment were acquired by large for-profit firms who restructured the services. This rapid set of transitions in health care delivery suggests a need to broadly assess the market in the following five force frameworks.

Force 1. Degree of Rivalry: Market Forces An industry analysis often focuses on a profile of the other providers in the area or region and stops there. The more focused the area providers are in their own areas of expertise, the more likely it is that they will recognize their interdependence and limit their rivalry.

In markets where several providers in the area seem to dominate, the group of similar providers tend to focus more on one another as they assess the market. This is typical of markets with one or more tertiary centers surrounded by community hospitals: The providers tend to only study their direct counterparts, when they should be comparing themselves to the highly differentiated and dominant provider. Only in recent years, with the heightened interest in affiliating with primary care providers to retain more market share and covered lives directly, has the rivalry circle grown to encompass any similar organization with the same type of services.

Because hospitals are so capital intensive and need a high level of utilization, price competition is a strong factor in market position. The right price of service may lead to more volume directed from the payers. Higher fixed costs, excess capacity, and lack of differentiation all lead to more intense rivalry. Hospitals have tried to differentiate themselves, with the result that consumers most often make physician and hospital selection decisions based on amenities—especially on self-referring services such as maternity care.

The extent of rivalry is determined by the diversity of the industry's goals and the risks of a strategic position. The less diverse the goals and the higher the stakes, the higher is the degree of rivalry. Markets with multiple similar providers, in which one is willing to make dramatic payer deals (50 percent discounted rates) for incremental volume, are touted as having an extremely high degree of rivalry. The marketplace may be unbalanced, but one provider's physicians and hospital beds are busy in the short term. In addition, when branded services that cannot be imitated are held by geographic franchise, there is little threat of substitutes across a geographic area.

Force 2. Threat of Entry: Potential Industry Players The most frequent forms of entry barriers are the scale and investment to enter an industry as an efficient competitor. Historically, the Determination/ Certificate-of-Need Process, as a state-administered program reviewing new services, provided regulatory barriers to entering a new service line market.

Health care organizations frequently rely on required regulatory agency reports to gain information on other providers. However, for-profit companies that are hiring physicians and managing practices are not subject to state licensing authorities. Therefore, tracking other players in the industry is a matter for both formal and informal information gathering.

Market research is an essential aid to track the consumer's preferences and physician selection criteria, key elements in understanding potential industry players. In addition, research is important to the providers of services. A new player in the market will need information in order to approach the market and existing players will want to monitor their own market to maintain their strategic position. An organization that knows what the customer wants will be able to forestall a potential player that may have neither the resources nor the time to both effectively introduce a competing service and induce consumers to switch. In addition to government sources, several industry sources of data on industry players, such as HCIA/Mercer and The Sachs Group, keep extensive databases.

Force 3. Threat of Substitutes: Potential Industry Players Substitution occurs where there is a product or service that can meet the same need as the existing product or service. As both clinical and managerial technology move ahead at a rapid rate, innovations in providing alternative diagnostic, treatment, or managerial options can provide a substitution for traditionally rendered services.

All services are composed of both core and augmented elements. The core of the health care provider services, the patient-physician relationship, has some (though few) substitutes, principally extending to specialists overseeing chronic conditions. However, the means of the physician's diagnosis and subsequent treatment plan has many capable substitutes. More and more, clinical technology can replace current means of diagnosis and treatment. Computer-aided diagnostic systems, while saving physician time and work, also, to a certain extent, serve as a substitute for direct patient time over a patient chart.

Other components of traditional patient-physician relationships, such as health education, diagnostic tests, and treatment options, are all open to substitution. Particularly in an era where physicians are being incited to increase patient bases, this ability to shift services to the least-cost provider is even more important and prevalent. Traditional health care providers could be relieved of providing augmented services—health education, counseling, lifestyle management, and cost information—and could concentrate on increasing panels of patients.

Health care services are already using substitutes in the following way:

- physician office management protocols instead of hospitalization
- new drug treatments replacing surgery
- new drug treatments replacing hospitalization
- minimally invasive procedures replacing more invasive treatment
- generic drugs lowering the cost of treatment
- alternative or complementary health care services replacing traditional medical care

Force 4. Buyer Power: Existing Industry Players Health care provider buyers command a lot of attention. The history of recommended health care reform options includes regulating the formation of health alliances that contract for federal health care dollars. The longer history of Medicare since the Nixon administration has established risk contracts that have been increasingly encouraged in recent years. Buyers have even greater leverage when buying as a coalition. The buyer may represent a high proportion of volume, such as the payer that dominates the market for managed care and contracts for the highest volume.

Health care coalitions of businesses, purchasing health care services together or sharing information systems to move ahead in purchasing, are another example of buyer power. Payers, also buyers of services, have moved into the health care delivery market as a means of getting market share. Buyers have the power to develop their own services to enter the market. The buyer poses a threat of backward integration, in which both payers and hospitals develop their own physician network system, controlling physician employment and practice management.

The payer who purchases a great deal of business is the most important customer to the health care delivery network, which is then vulnerable to the moves of one organization. Making changes to satisfy a major customer may make the organization unsuitable to others in the marketplace, and therefore more vulnerable and more dependent. For example, when a hospital's dominant payer is one managed care firm, the hospital threatens the loss of that volume when making unfriendly moves to ally with another payer. The timetable for getting enrollees to switch payers in order to maintain the provider affiliation may be a lot shorter than is thought.

Finally, the services provided by each health care organization may not be sufficiently differentiated. Market research is necessary to check the consumer's or the payer's perspective and willingness to switch. If there is not sufficient differentiation between industry players, consumers or buyers who cannot determine a good enough reason not to switch will change health care delivery providers easily.

Force 5. Supplier Power: Existing Industry Players Suppliers influence the health care provider industry by setting prices based on more than just the cost of supplies. The acute care provider industry is heavily regulated, and the payer industry is informally regulated by heavy publicity. On the other hand, the nonregulated supplier industry seems to have an easy hand in price setting, based on the patent of technology. Technology is not always replicable, although providers moving to standardization of service delivery are less reliant on brand technology than in the past.

To the extent that health care delivery organizations seek cost efficiency though bidding, the power of suppliers is more reliant on technology and drugs that are protected by patents. In those businesses, the purchase is made of specific products. However, in the case of specific technologies (like aggressive fertility treatment) or specific drugs (like nongeneric brands), payers pass the costs to the consumer either directly, by refusing to cover those services or drugs, or indirectly, by increasing the consumer portion of payment.

FRAMEWORKS FOR ASSESSING THE HEALTH CARE INDUSTRY

To effectively complete one or more of the industry analytic models described previously, the following frameworks can be used to place the analytic tools and their results in a health care context:

- national trends
- industry arena identification
- health care delivery models
- internal/organizational assessment
- payer position assessment
- market position assessment
- geographic assessment

These frameworks are discussed in the following subsections.

National Trends

Several categories of activities should be watched when assessing national trends for policy and statistical performance. Organizations in leading-edge states tend to respond more quickly to market forces. For example, Minnesota (especially the Twin Cities area) has a reputation for being a more advanced market concerning managed care and integrated systems development. California represents a more advanced physician group consolidation market. Illinois (especially the Chicago area) represents a market with advanced affiliations. Each of these markets has learned lessons from which other organizations can benefit.

In addition, annual environmental updates are issued by industry groups and think tanks. These regular updates are essential, as many national research groups conclude that information can quickly become dated—many assumptions apply only to factors in the stated time period. In the absence of national reform, industry analyses incorporate new data from different areas; staying current is critical to responding to the free market system.

Industry updates cover a wide range of issues relative to the merging industries of payer and provider. The best advice is to keep current with several expert updates. Sources for industry updates include criteria for investment, trade groups, professional groups, and health care consulting firms (which have their own industry updates). At a minimum, review the following types of materials:

- publications from think tanks or public or private research companies that examine key issues and trends
- models from other "mature" areas (for instance, Minnesota or California)
- information regarding environmental change in other locations
- expertise from futurists' research and consulting
- experiences of progressive companies that nationally move in payer circles, purchaser coalitions, and provider networks
- private investment funds that support innovations in health care
- national forum topics—what the providers, payers, and futurists are saying

Industry Arena Identification

Given the larger context of the environment in which this industry exists, the analysis of the health care industry has to be focused more globally than locally. Health care delivery services operate in three main industry arenas:

1. health care prevention and maintenance
2. medical service delivery
3. postservice delivery support services

Most health care organizations also function to some extent in the payer side of the service delivery system.

Industry Components of the Service Delivery System   Table 3-2 identifies industry components of the service delivery system. Once in the system, care is provided for prevention and early diagnosis, primary care, hospital care, specialty care, and postspecialty and hospital services.

Scope of Service Delivery   Thoroughly reviewing the scope of service delivery and the number of industries in which an organization participates will result in a more relevant industry assessment. The analysis may be based on a product category or a user benefit category. It is important not to define the industry categories too narrowly. Most organizations will look at the scope of all payers (all insurance companies) as well as all providers, along with a specific review of those that function in both arenas. Any health care organization may include the categories of activities listed in table 3-2. Therefore a clarification of the scope of services and products is necessary before deciding how the industry will be assessed.

Three traditional scopes—horizontal, vertical, and geographic—are commonly used to assess industry structures. When using this framework, an organization must decide whether to classify its structure into subcategories. For example, a health care organization with a payer component or direct contracting function could be profiled relative to the payer industry as well as to the payer and provider industry. The definition of industry boundaries remains as much an art as a science, with most of the ambiguities involving various dimensions of scope.[7]

Horizontal scope: This scope of assessment spans across product specific markets. The advantage of this approach is that a product-specific analysis will reveal information that might benefit both a particular product and an organization's strategic position. However, looking only at comparable services may rule out potential entrance into a market. With strong financial reserves, an organization could enter the market faster than a typical health care organization that must develop a similar "war chest." For example, if every area organization was assessed as a potential purchaser of physician practices, then more potential industry participants would be apparent. Until recently, payers would not have been expected to be a provider of both physicians and hospitals. Yet throughout the country, payers have moved toward gaining access to the insurance enrollees who make insurance and provider decisions in tandem by developing provider services.

Vertical scope: This scope of assessment encompasses the continuum of care. Although diversification focused on developing cradle-to-grave services to provide an entire health care system, vertical integration of care continues for other purposes. The expected onset of capitation as the dominant reimbursement mechanism for providers should reinforce vertical

TABLE 3-2. Health Care Industry Components

Patient Access to Provider System	Prevention and Early Diagnosis	Primary Care	Hospital Care	Specialty Care	Postspecialty and Hospital Services
Access to insurance and payer products	Health education and outreach	Targeted health education through self-management manuals and written instruction, videos, and self-management support services	Ancillary and hospital-based physician services	Referral criteria management and utilization review	Follow-up support of clinical service delivery and monitoring pathways
Payer copayments and deductibles	Health testing and screening	Telephone support services prior to care	Emergency care—criteria for services	Specialty care physician services	Home care and support services during recovery
Payer approved providers and services	Inoculations	Primary care physician services with physician extenders	Observation care—criteria for services		Social support services
	Drug compliance	After-hours care	Acute admission care		Nursing home or supervised living
	Social management for high-risk groups				

integration. Capitation suggests that providers will develop the capacity for the continuum of care to enhance efficiency and lower costs. This view is tempered by cautions of conventional wisdom that virtual integration precedes the complicated work of acquisition and merger—that is, there is real form to the function of integration. Both suppliers and purchasers have opportunities for cooperative as well as competitive behavior. The potential partnership with purchasers or suppliers enables savings on overhead expenses and efficiencies in cost and operation that may benefit the participating organizations and the health care systems themselves. The necessary first step to such a consideration is to assess the available services inherent in vertical integration.

Geographic scope: This assessment covers the geographic service areas, or service area reach of services and products. Although health care delivery system service areas have generally been local, the development of satellites—notably by the Cleveland Clinic and the Mayo Clinic—in other parts of the country has changed all that. The integration of health care delivery systems across greater geographic areas in search of more covered lives and a larger patient base also has broadened the marketplace for most providers. The Blue Cross/Blue Shield companies in New England have announced intentions to work together to ensure access to care. In such a small area, employees in one state may live in another. Similarly, health care delivery systems located near state borders must include organizations in other states—despite their differences in data—to assess the service area accurately.

Health Care Delivery Models

Although health care delivery services are largely viewed as businesses serving local constituents, the reach of national resources—such as management firms and certain payers—makes it more of a nationally based and locally focused industry. Because the industry drivers are national in scope and locally specific, models of the industry operations show both the range of variation and the potential next steps for change. There have been several models developed by industry experts for assessing the managed care marketplace. Consumers use different criteria in selecting their payers, depending on the choices and levels of care that are offered.

In 1995, The Sachs Group conducted research in 27 markets and provided models and insight into how consumers' attitudes and behavior have changed as managed care has matured. They found that cost and convenience alone do not guarantee the selection of a plan; secondary factors influence selections. Those secondary factors differ by market stage and by market. In growing markets, product and cost differentiation drive plan selection, but they are less important in mature markets.[8] (See tables 3-3 and 3-4.)

In 1994, VHA issued a report on "Integration: Market Forces and Critical Success Factors," using the experiences of VHA institutions involved in integrated health care system development. In a review of market factors, it was found that markets differed but can be characterized by four market stages, each with its own delivery system expectations. Each stage is fundamentally different from the preceding one in terms of expectations about market price; degrees of physical, operational, and clinical integration; and the preference for provider integration. It is

TABLE 3-3. Market Evolution Model and Managed Care Product Life Cycles

Characteristic	Stage I	Stage II	Stage III	Stage IV
Type of Managed Care Market	Unstructured market	Loose, fragmented market	Consolidating market	Tight market
Degree of Managed Care	Little managed care penetration	Growing managed care presence	Increasingly competitive managed care market; tightening utilization	Very competitive; consolidation of plans; tight utilization control
Place in the Industry Cycle	Immature, young market	Growth market	Maturing market	Mature market

Source: Sachs Group, adapted from University HealthSystem Consortium (UHC).

TABLE 3-4. Retention and Acquisition Strategies

	Stage II	Stage III	Stage IV
Membership Strategy	Increase market size through acquisition of new enrollees	Stabilize position through retention and acquisition	Increase and stabilize leadership position; retain and steal market share
Network Strategy	Develop network	Solidify network	Develop network for niche marketing
Promotional Focus	Emphasize familiarity of name, physicians, and hospitals	Product differentiation, favorable evaluations, better benefits	Product extensions, niche marketing, building on brand equity
Marketing Message	"New delivery; same quality"	"Better than the rest"	"We're not just a health plan"

Source: Sachs Group.

notable that stage IV represents an expected future state for the most sophisticated marketplaces but that none had reached this stage at the time the model was developed.[9] (See figure 3-1.)

Internal Organizational Assessment

An internal evaluation, including specific details, is the first requirement of any organizational strategic assessment. This assessment can be completed in conjunction with one of the industry analysis models described earlier in the chapter. Understanding the external environment, although extremely important, can only be valuable in the context of understanding the organization's internal capabilities. The assessment should be maintained on a regular basis to avoid strategic surprises, to identify emerging issues, and to resolve problems before they escalate. Although operating data are likely to be contained in any of several departments or areas, the most important component is that the information be available to the management team and assessed regularly.

FIGURE 3-1. Market Stages

Stage I	*Stage III*
Convenience	Market defines price
No limits	Excess capacity eliminated from payments
Choice	
Fragmented	Market demands "real" managed care
Absolute professional model	
Discounting	Market demands exclusivity
Beginning of purchaser (employer) involvement	Market demands a longitudinal perspective
Beginning of physician "anxiety" (the world may change)	*Stage IV*
Solo practice still viable	Accountable for quality, service, access
Stage II	Accountable for health status
Per-capita cost (price) of care matters	Some limits to intervention
Overcapacity still exists (prevails)	Full purchaser market power
• Specialists	Incentives to do the "wrong thing" are eliminated
• Hospitals (some reduction)	
Some market power of purchaser	
Beginning of exclusivity	
Consolidating physician organizations (small solo marginally viable)	
Highly "anxious" physicians	

The ability to analyze an organization's performance internally becomes essential in payer contracts, in public demonstration of value or differentiation, and in setting objectives to enhance or modify specific areas requiring attention. Issues to analyze should be defined first. Once they are defined and the relevant data are identified, the issues should be compared and evaluated against one another. A rank ordering should be developed to depict how an organization compares to its own prior years' findings, to other organizations in the system, and to other organizations selected for comparison. Several excellent software programs—which an organization may already have or may purchase from a consultant—have this capability. Many database systems contain analysis-ready algorithms and comparative features that can incorporate organizational data and formulate various types of reports.

Internal assessment should focus on the following key areas:

- clinical activity and performance
- medical staff
- financial position
- payer position

Clinical Activity and Performance Assessment Clinical information such as occupancy rates, market share, and so on can be used to profile an organization. This information can be detailed by such operating areas as acute, subacute, ambulatory, and home care. Determining clinical activity and performance generates the internal assessment, showing strengths and weaknesses in a clinical management context. This assessment may suggest frameworks for management of clinical operations and indicate objectives that need to be developed during the strategic assessment.

Physician Assessment The affiliated physician assessment is the first step in understanding the medical community. For instance, the staff representation may show a surplus of specialists compared to primary care providers. Comparing contracted physicians and nonaffiliated physicians to the target market can result in a decision either to add volume or types of providers in a geographically balanced fashion. The age profile may suggest planned replacements based on who is retiring.

Knowing what providers are available, compared to what providers are needed—and when—helps shape decisions on contracts. For example, one health care organization that noted diminishing admissions from a physician group found that it was seriously affected by that group's negotiations for purchase by a for-profit physician practice company. The physicians realized that the purchase price would be based on office revenue, and the physicians sought to maximize that revenue to raise the purchase price. Monitoring and a direct discussion with the physician group likely would have identified the potential change sooner.

Financial Position Assessment The financial position assessment should compare costs and fees with other providers and identify areas that contribute to the higher costs in key clinical departments or services. Further, identifying either available capital or capital needs is important to assess the ability to fund strategic priorities and achieve strategic outcomes. The following cost ratios should be computed for this analysis:

- average cost per discharge
- average cost per stay
- operating margin
- day's cash on hand
- debt service coverage
- return on assets

The results will show operating efficiencies for the organization under review as compared to itself and its competitors.

Payer Position Assessment Understanding your targeted marketplace from the payers' viewpoint will help develop a payer position. Payer position issues may include targeting the level of covered lives cared for in the health care system; determining who is affiliated with the primary care providers; discovering if the covered lives exceed the capacity of the primary care providers; or determining whether there is a shortage in any of a number of areas, based on the geographic distribution or age distribution of the medical staff. Payer position assessments should measure the following:

- active markets
- utilization of plan by group
- enrollees by product line
- primary care provider locations
- financial indicators
- employer lists
- list of contracting providers
- days per 1,000 by product line

A marketplace payer should be assessed in terms of what it can offer, what it does offer, and what its relationship is and could be with the organization. A trend assessment of payers operating in other markets can help an organization determine its own potential position in a new market. Regional payers, who may be anticipating expansion into the local market, also should be assessed for their strengths, weaknesses, and relationship potential. In addition, relationships with other providers are important indicators about potential payers. Specifically, a payer's relationships with acute care facilities and physicians are critical in considering whether an organization should pursue a relationship enhancement with that payer. For instance, a payer who involves physicians in setting fees is going to be a very different kind of partner than one who changes fee schedules unilaterally.

An assessment of marketplace payers should study

- all contracts
- payer contract buyers
- physician preferences in payer contract criteria
- options for physician-hospital contracting

Contract assessment: Contract assessment is useful to review both stated and effective contract terms. Differences may exist, based on the variables in each contract and, for multiple year contracts, in the expected and actual payment rates. For example, if payment terms are based on case mix intensity, effective payment rates may be greater or less than budgeted levels. A contract assessment would review the contract payment terms, effective payment terms, contract length, clinical service definitions, and termination option by payer contract. This assessment would check for variability and surprises in the contracts compared to expected performance. Contract requirements should include meeting financial requirements for the organization and terms for clinical management of patients, such as payment for emergency visits for people with life-threatening symptoms. An organization should look for opportunities to improve the payer position and the means of acquiring larger groups of patients.

Contract buyer assessment: The goals of the payers are a function of the regional marketplace, payer interest in obtaining employer accounts, and payer desire to increase enrollment in each account. These goals and interests are based on their current versus their preferred contracting position. Knowing the employers' preferences in the marketplace is essential in constructing a payer platform. The employers' valuing of information and perception of provider information are relevant to how they will be approached by payers, and their contracts will subsequently affect providers. The same assessment should be done for government purchasers of health care services. The extent of risk in Medicare contracts has an impact on the payer platform. Medicaid contracting criteria also impact the payer platform.

Physician preference assessment: Physicians in private practice have opinions and preferences about payers, their terms, the way fees are set, and the way utilization is managed. These opinions and preferences must be researched and, if possible, a consensus developed about contracting. The physicians, to the extent that preferences are shared, may wish to join together as a physician group or with the hospital to develop a contract. The primary care physicians and the specialists are likely to have separate issues and agendas. However, it is essential to articulate the position of the physicians and to consider the options for developing a shared contracting vehicle to simplify contracting, if that is relevant to the payers. Ultimately, if a group is formed, allocation of fees must be part of the contract.

Options for physician contracting assessment: Both physician participation and leadership are essential in moving ahead as either a larger physician group or as a health care delivery system. Participants in a health care delivery network may comprise both existing physicians and supplemental physicians (for practice growth, if there is a demonstrated need). Goals should be established to address physician relationships within a large group, within a health care delivery system, and in response to managing care for a specific population or a set of payer contracts.

Physician group structures: A variety of structures enable physicians to work together and health care delivery systems to work with physicians—with ranges of autonomy, access to resources, and means of coming together.

- *Physician–hospital organization (PHO):* A PHO is a legal entity formed by a hospital and a group of physicians to further mutual interests and to achieve market objectives. A PHO generally combines physicians and a hospital into a single provider organization for the purpose of obtaining managed care contracts.
- *Management services organization (MSO):* An MSO is a legal entity that provides administrative and management services to physicians—including managed care contracting services—and that may purchase the assets of physicians' practices.
- *Independent practice association (IPA):* An IPA can comprise individual physicians and group practices. An IPA negotiates and administers managed care contracts for its members. The physician members may share risks and profits from capitated payments for physician primary care and, under some contracts, for specialty care and hospital services.
- *Affiliated medical practice corporation (AMPC):* An AMPC is a tax-exempt corporation usually established under the umbrella of a hospital's holding company. An AMPC employs physicians to provide medical services to patients in the hospital's service area.

Physicians seeking contracts with one another or with a hospital should consider a number of issues, including the following:

- capital financing
- physician or hospital members arrangement composition
- number of physicians
- open and closed physician-hospital arrangements
- physician practice acquisitions

The primary care provider–specialist mix: The more that insurance products require primary care gatekeepers, the greater the need for primary care providers in a marketplace. This need shifts the focus from specialists (who have generated more revenue) to primary care providers (who have generated less revenue but are essential to adding covered lives to a system). No health care organization can survive without an appropriate mix of specialist physicians and primary care providers.

Thus, the successful future of health care systems or communities depends on primary care services. The greater demand for primary care providers has encouraged specialty-trained physicians to perform primary care; health care organizations are also amassing reserve funds to buy or create primary care practices. Most academic medical centers and even community hospitals have more specialists than primary care physicians.

The correct mix of primary care providers and specialists depends on the marketplace; the more managed care, the greater the need for primary care physicians. Increasingly, community hospitals and satellite facilities are developing primary care residency programs that allow the tertiary hospital to present itself in a new light. This change is part of the shift from acute care service delivery to primary care service delivery, supported by an appropriate mix of specialists.

The available mix of physicians to provide care for a population or group of covered lives should be assessed based on market share, as well as on actual and potential contracts. Some organizational designs call for an equal ratio of primary care physicians to specialists. What appears to be an equal mix, however, may be an illusion: In fact, many specialists provide both specialty and primary care, the latter as a supplement to their practices and in response to patients' requests. Assessment also should consider the productivity and panel sizes for each of the primary care physicians. Small panel sizes require more physicians to cover a group of covered lives.

Market Position Assessment

The market assessment focuses on the applicable definition of the area served by the organization. Ellen F. Goldman and Kevin C. Nolan point out that health care, like politics, is local.[10] Although national employers may buy health care coverage across the country, even national providers that operate in multiple markets must tailor their strategy to the local market. For example, Tenet takes a local approach to provider management. Edward Tudanger, senior vice president of operations for the southeast region of Tenet Health Care Corporation, has said, "The strategic issues revolve around one key question: How can this hospital ensure a healthy future for itself so that it can continue to provide needed care to the community? The answers vary—hospital by hospital, community by community, and deal by deal."[11]

In order to better assess the market position of the organization in each of its service areas, a number of factors should be considered:

- characteristics of the population living and working in each service area
- market share (whether the organization is a leader, if market share is increasing or decreasing, and the organization's market presence over several years)
- customer assessment (whom the organization serves)
- competitor assessment

Population Characteristics The populations living in each of the service areas have likely changed with economic development or decline. Both the total and the parts of the service areas offer opportunities to analyze the population of those living in the area. Comparing key demographic trends to prior years, and identifying key needs by the clusters of households, provides indicators of services that would be needed for health care delivery organizations. A market share and demographic analysis should review the following:

- market share by city or town (indicates where the organization has the strongest market presence)
- patient origin by city or town (indicates where patients are from and shows any increases or decreases by area)
- population cohorts by age, gender, origin (nationality), and geographic location (indicates potential for tailoring services and forecasting upcoming needs such as elderly care)
- education level and average household income (indicate health status)
- employment by type and distance from home (indicate health status)

Expert demographic analysis and demographic databases are helpful tools in identifying population characteristics. Trends in demography, observed by the local town and city governments, the health boards' data on health issues, and population trends provide valuable information.

Identifying new population groups: Identification of new population groups may be evidenced more by civic government than by the update of national demographic information. Realtors can also point to significant changes in housing: The extent to which area residents work in the same area where they live, work outside the area where they live, or work in the area but live elsewhere, has important contributing factors to health care services.

For example, a suburban staff model HMO developed a site outside a major city and forecast the enrollees that the primary care site would accommodate. The actual enrollment was nearly double that of the anticipated enrollment because the site was located near a well-traveled public transit line. People who traveled on that transit line decided to get their health care services on the way to and from work, rather than close to one site or another.

Key public health issues can also be revealed by studies of public health indicators, new populations, and the presence and services for new populations such as ethnic groups who may have limited access to health care.

Assessing the correct service mix: The demographic profile should be compared to available services to ensure a correct mix. Although it may appear to be an appropriate mix of services, further assessment would refine both the actual services offered and the service access provided. For example, the cultural barriers for some populations are worth evaluating to ensure appropriate access. On a simpler basis, working parents would likely prefer pediatricians and family practitioners who offered evening and weekend hours and adult medical care with the same access.

Market Share   Ideally, a health care organization should answer the following questions about its service areas:

- Where are patients coming from?
- Where are patients in the service area going to obtain health care?
- In the case of market share increase or decrease, what other providers(s) have had the opposite increase or decrease, potentially accounting for the patterns of use of health care providers?
- What is the key point of differentiation between the organization and the other major providers, and which has demonstrated weaknesses and strengths?

Collecting market share data: The collection of market share data requires a database that provides information about other providers serving comparable regions. Some states—including Minnesota, Massachusetts, and Rhode Island—require hospitals and health care systems to provide data relating to admissions, emergency department utilization, and other types of utilization information. However, in other states, the market position has to be estimated in other ways.

An organization's market position would first provide the market share information by clinical service, by DRG, by payer, by length of stay (LOS), by charge, and by age/sex population groups. Then comparisons can be made of the performance over the last three to five years. This information should be used to look for trends within each key area, to identify other providers serving that market in terms of major players, and to identify peripheral players. In addition, the data can help identify tertiary providers who attract both self-referred patients and community provider referrals. Tertiary providers seeking to increase market share may well take advantage of a tertiary referral position and a self-referring population to place primary care providers into the marketplace.

Considering utilization: Market share information focuses on the inpatient hospital discharges for hospitals and enrollees. This was more valid as an indicator of hospital encounters before the substitutes for inpatient medicine (observation care rather than short-stay admissions; ambulatory surgery instead of inpatient surgery) became so prevalent. Although many states have centralized hospital discharge databases for market share analysis, most have not replicated that level of information for these alternatives to hospital inpatient care. Thus only some organizations (such as health plans or physician groups) have this information—which is quite limited compared to the marketwide information previously available.

Market share analysis thus requires both consideration of the offsetting observation cases and ambulatory surgery cases that have become substitutes for hospital encounters. In addition, utilization figures have nationally shown a decline in admissions for most populations because of alternative treatment modalities. Therefore, measuring market share as an absolute figure, without considering utilization, would be a mistake.

Customers and Their Needs In addition to identifying and assessing various aspects of the health care industry, organizations must consider various customers and their needs. Customers have traditionally been identified through medical staff physicians, on whom the hospital relied for admissions. During the last two decades, strategies were instituted to increase physician bonding with patients in order to win the loyalty of those admitted to multiple hospitals. Physicians have also been encouraged to align more closely with the health care organization. Providers also used increased direct promotion and decreased pricing to attract payer contracts.

Organizations used traditional marketing activities in program design: pricing to get and keep payer contracts, and establishing self-referred primary care services (both primary care providers and maternity service) where geographically desired. Efforts aimed at aggressively promoting service to draw consumers to the self-refer services have been through many iterations. Abandoning traditional reliance on physicians, these efforts are moving toward managing relationships with many of the end-users of the health care delivery organization. This effort requires moving from the traditional strategies toward emphases on consumer sales, industrial products, and, finally, relationship management.

An organization should complete the following steps to understand its relationship with its customers:

1. Identify all customer groups involved in the purchase decision(s) to attract customers.
2. Assess all the choices that those customers have in making the specific component of the decision.
3. Identify the ease of making different decisions.
4. Identify ways of decreasing the cost of making different selection decisions.
5. Develop industrial-type contracts that keep customers tied to the service in the long run.
6. Build a positive image to encourage the selection decision.
7. Continue to recognize other choices that each customer group can make and track the factors involved in those choices.

Customer groups: Customer groups comprise all participants in the health care service delivery selection. The groups involved in the purchase decision to attract health care customers include:

- self-refer specialists (for instance, obstetrician/gynecologists)
- specialist physicians
- payers
- public programs (Medicare/Medicaid) that select the payer
- employers that select the payer
- employees
- family members of employees

Building databases on customer groups: Each customer group can play a role in the individual customer's decision about where to obtain health care services. Building a database about each of the groups in the customer base is important: This information is used to conduct market research through individual interviews, either directly or through an intermediary (a consultant), focus groups, and surveys (written or telephone). The focus of the market research is to gather information about customers' current situations, the pressures facing them, and their interests in developing and maintaining a long-term relationship with a health care institution. Market research can be used to evaluate the following:

- *Payers:* Payers can be evaluated by building a database and by conducting interviews. A third party is recommended for conducting interviews, because criticism can be expressed with less bias. In addition, the options for discussion, which may be brainstorming, are not interpreted as negotiations when an outside party, like a consultant, is involved.
- *Employers or employer purchasing groups:* Interviews or surveys are useful methods for evaluating these groups. Employers can identify the health care organization's clinical volume and net revenue. Questions should be asked about current and preferred payer relationships for health care organizations that lack a financing component. Such indirect relationships may result in more direct communication between the provider and employer.
- *Public programs:* This evaluation is similar to that of employer or employer purchasing groups, except that public programs (Medicare/Medicaid) are buying private payer products (such as risk contracts). Thus the organization should assess both the current private/public program (managed Medicaid, managed Medicare volumes), as well as the nonmanaged public program participation (volume and revenue for Medicare and Medicaid patients and the last several years of trends in those populations).

Selective contracting based on price locks out patients and can encourage switching. For short-term (such as annual) or easy-out contracts, the provider list can change as easily as the termination clause. Partnerships may ensure a longer term relationship, but the value to the employer is then based only on price. Even if employers move to low cost health plans, the decision to limit the access based only on cost may alienate consumer choice and threaten employee relationships.

Evaluating the interests of the area residents suggests qualitative and quantitative market research to identify and point out key attributes of the current service delivery, the means of selection, and the preferred provider selection and payer selection. With "hard to reach" groups, qualitative research (focus groups, interviews) may be helpful in identifying means of gathering more information about serving special groups such as seniors, specific ethnic populations, or persons with disabilities.

Assessing customer groups: Assessment of all customer groups (patients, enrollees, physicians, and payers) is essential to determine the stage of market level of integration and control, and to develop direction for the future. Knowing what influences local decision making and what is important to local customer groups better equips the health care institution to develop needed and desired products and services.

The assessment of choices that each customer group has in selecting a health care organization is influenced by the primary care provider. Identify where the office is located, to what organization they admit their patients (and why), and what would persuade the physician to switch or maintain his or her loyalty.

Under fee-for-service arrangements, customers have more choices about where to go for health care. Under managed care, those choices may be more restrictive, based on the rules of the payer. Therefore, it is important to gauge choices open to various customer groups.

Preferred tertiary institutions for community hospital physicians should be identified. In the 1980s, physicians outside tertiary hospitals referred patients to tertiary hospitals based on one of two factors: either where they trained or where they knew tertiary physicians and were comfortable about the way their referrals were received. Market research is the best determinant to assess the referring patterns and criteria.

For employed people, check other insurer options by employer. Premiums, copayments, provider access, or exclusions are indications of what may be appealing to employees. The rate structure for single persons, families, and two adults is important to know.

Geographic Assessment

The categorization of strategic data can revolve around a pictorial image of the health care organization and its service area. Figure 3-2 depicts the geographic scope of a health care organization's database. From the smallest locus of service operation to the largest, the circles in figure 3-2 are drawn to start with the health care organization itself, moving to the primary service area, and further broadening the information base to the national level. The service area is the geographic area served by the organization: (1) primary service area, (2) secondary service area, and (3) tertiary service area (statewide and nationwide).

Primary Service Area With the hospital at the planning core, the first geographic level to evaluate is the primary service area. The primary service area refers to the towns and cities that account for 80 to 90 percent of the hospital's market share. The opportunity for collaboration lies in service provision for acute and nonacute service providers. Anyone providing services to that marketplace may be appropriate for collaboration in service planning.

The majority of the patients cared for live in this collection of towns and cities, because they take advantage of the easiest access. However, as the

FIGURE 3-2. Geographic Scope of a Health Care Organization Database

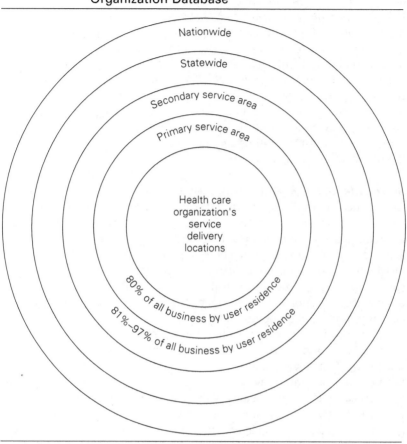

core definition of clinical care shifts from inpatient to outpatient, and the inpatient status is divided among subacute care services as well as observation status, a greater mix of patient status will be used in identifying the service area. The identification of the market position—based on market share data—will follow the identification of the service area. Most important, the compelling health status needs of the local population must be identified.

Secondary Service Area The secondary service area is composed of the towns and cities that are often adjacent to the health care provider's primary service area. This area makes up the smaller proportion of a hospital's admissions and represents patients who are drawn to a health care provider, despite a greater distance traveled, for some type of specialty or differentiated services. The secondary service area draw may be due to a few specialty services rather than an overall examination of primary care access services. This broader service area is the focus for identifying other providers with which to share equipment (for instance, mobile MRIs) and specialists or the range of specialists requiring more than one hospital for their specialty (for instance, infectious disease specialists).

Generally, from 10 percent to 20 percent of the patients are from this collection of towns and cities. This is identified from the list of the annual inpatient and outpatient customers. Secondary service area information can be profiled by provider, payer, and demography. The conclusions from the secondary service area assessment may note whether markets are worth moving into from a secondary or tertiary position, or if there is merit in establishing outposts in the secondary service area to broaden the primary service area.

Statewide Service Area This service area includes the towns and cities outside both the health care provider's primary and secondary service areas. This tier is the focus for identifying other providers with which to share participation in insurance and group purchasing. Proximity allows some similarity in product development. The statewide area is one in which collaboration for policy and information with other providers can allow an organization to respond to regulations, market share, or other data collection efforts through standardization of reporting. It is also important for competitor analyses.

The draw from this area is often for a specific service that other area providers do not offer. An example of a statewide service area reach is a transplant or invasive clinical services (not offered in specific places). Each tertiary program may have its unique service area draw and, more specifically, specialty physicians with their own key referral sources that make up the service area draw. These service area draws are unrelated to the majority of care provided by the rest of the organization. Most tertiary hospitals draw from within one hundred miles. However, the proclivity to have a tertiary service area can be based on referral patterns of known referrers, brand name, and reputation.

Nationwide Service Area The final area is the national scope, which offers a number of opportunities for providers. For instance, providers can collaborate for information on national policy, form alliances in non-competing markets, share data projects, and even extend their purchasing group alliance.

APPROACH TO AFFILIATION

Collaborative partner selection can be complicated. Selecting an agency or service with which to collaborate is an essential part of planning. It is important to develop criteria with which to regard the potential affiliations. Affiliations based on concepts founded in abstracted literature reviews cannot replace the clarification of operating priorities for the health care organization. Development of these priorities and the subsequent criteria list will enable an affiliate shopping excursion to be a meaningful way to establish organizational advantages.

Understanding the Goals of Affiliation

The conclusions from an environmental analysis should identify how an organization is serving the marketplace as well as what other capabilities would improve its strategic position. For example, if an organization needs certain benefits to hold the desired market position, but has neither the resources nor time to develop them from scratch, an organization holding that position would be an excellent ally. If a geographic market is growing, an opportunity to provide services may be most expeditiously done with an affiliation. Another provider or payer with expertise in prepaid Medicare or Medicaid may offer a potential affiliation to share those core competencies.

It is important for the organization to understand the goal of the collaboration. Possible goals for collaborative ventures can include the following:

- to make concrete inroads to become a system with demonstrable benefits
- to explore affiliation options to fit the vision of the organization, without forgoing nonprofit status or health- or service-related provisions.
- to demonstrate to payers and employers the value of the organization in response to broad-based concerns over health care costs
- to respond to the proposals for health reform, including prepaid government contracts (Medicare/Medicaid)

This understanding needs reach both service- and product-specific levels.

Identifying the Added Value of Affiliation

Identifying the added value that the collaboration provides is another important element of these goals. An assessment of the hospital's strengths and weaknesses, as well as the possible affiliate's strengths and weaknesses, enhances the ability to have equal or comparable partnership in a venture. This assessment should include the financial strength of each player. The benefit to the patient and client in collaboration is another key element to this equation. Understanding each player's access to consumers, patients, and clients (and who has access) rounds out the key elements to address in collaborative partner selection.

Collaboration opportunities should focus on the following sets of potential purposes:

- enhanced services offerings
- expanded referral sources
- improved images
- economies of scale
- capacity to structure delivery system and allocate resources
- improved access to capital
- improved debt capacity
- integration of all essential systems elements (underwriting, provision of services, and administration)
- allowance for a systems approach to care delivery, utilization review, resource allocation, and pricing
- allowance for flexibility in pricing and service arrangements
- hospital or PHO control of system
- primacy of provider perspective in formation of system

LESSONS LEARNED FROM PERFORMING ENVIRONMENTAL ANALYSES

The environmental analysis provides both conclusions about what is needed in the regional marketplace and the opportunities to impact those circumstances. Identifying organizations facing similar circumstances provides valuable timesaving opportunities to design appropriate tactics in order to move rapidly.

Innovations by other organizations, on a national or international level, often provide the best lessons and examples for the health care organization establishing its own directions. The variation of markets in service innovation, managed care maturity, and level of integration suggests that the local markets change quickly. Any organization can learn from others in and out of its own market.

Many avenues exist to educate various groups (physicians, managers, physician leaders) about the national scope of options in innovation, including the use of consultants and other expert resources. Whatever method is chosen, it is essential that the leaders of the organization benefit from others' successes and failures. Integration, payer relationships, and community health status can be used as a framework to assess success.

Mistakes in Integration

A review of industry experts, providers, and industry literature highlights the following challenges organizations face when approaching integration:

- No consensus is reached on the mission and vision.
- Linkages are developed without consistent objectives.
- Alliance does not anticipate the reaction of the other providers in the marketplace (competitors).
- Integration strategy development precedes the market assessment.
- Partners or collaborators are selected based on who is the most aggressive.

Mistakes in Payer Relationships

In consideration of payer relationships, the changes in provider-payer management require attention to the contracts, rather than to points of renewal. Successful contracts will depend on avoiding the following mistakes:

- Payer contracts are established without an assessment of the economic impact on the organization.
- There is disparity among payers.
- There is favorable incremental volume pricing without clarity about new or switched volume.
- Payer is not monitored (in such areas as payments, utilization changes, payments to physicians and incentives to physicians, market position, employer accounts).
- The organization fails to consider competitor reactions.

Mistakes in Community Health Status

The following mistakes have proven to be costly to those responding to community health status:

- Identification of resident health needs comes from demographic data only, rather than from market research.
- There is a widely held belief that the provider alone can make an impact.
- The organization responds to needs in terms of control rather than collaboration.
- The initiatives focus on the development of short-term interventions that cannot be sustained.

- The organization exclusively focuses on health care in response to health status issues.

These common mistakes are identified consistently by industry leaders and evident in recent health care literature. Avoiding these mistakes, while following the analytical steps identified in this chapter, can help an organization conquer the hurdles of strategic assessment and create a successful market strategy.[12]

CONCLUSION

Correctly assessing the business environment is critical for taking actions that are advantageous to the health care organization. The first step is to develop the list of industry drivers. That means looking at a number of overlapping and shifting factors, including economics, technology, politics, clinical treatment, and consumer requirements. Then, once the industry drivers have been analyzed and the market has been assessed, a strategy platform can be formulated to maximize opportunities on an objective basis. The range of directions may include partnerships as a tactical tool.

References

1. "Working Together to Shape the Future," *Environmental Assessment 93/94* (Chicago: American Society for Healthcare Marketing and Planning, 1994), p. 15.

2. "People of the Year," *HR Magazine,* vol. 41, no. 9 (Sept. 1996): 86.

3. Jeff Goldsmith, speech to the Annual Meeting of the Society for Healthcare Strategy and Market Development, September 1991.

4. S. Ghoshal and D. E. Westney, "Organizing Competitor Analysis Systems" *Strategic Management Journal* 12 (1991): pp. 17-31.

5. *Litchfield [Conn.] County Times,* June 30, 1995.

6. Michael E. Porter, *Competitive Strategy* (New York: The Free Press, 1980), p. 4.

7. David Collis and Pankaj Ghemawat, "Industry Analysis: Understanding Industry Structure and Dynamics," in *The Portable MBA in Strat-*

egy by Liam Fahey and Robert M. Randall (New York: Wiley, 1994), p. 175.

8. "The Road to Increased Market Share: Meeting Changing Consumer Expectations about Health Care" (Evanston, Ill.: Sachs Group, 1996.)

9. VHA Inc., "Integration: Market Forces and Critical Success Factors" (Irving, Tex.: VHA Inc., 1994), p. 23.

10. Ellen F. Goldman and Kevin C. Nolan, *Strategic Planning in Health Care: A Guide for Board Members* (Chicago: American Hospital Publishing, 1994), p. 8.

11. "Hometown Hospitals, National Resources," *Health Systems Review* (May/June 1997): pp. 28-29.

12. Gerry Johnson, "Strategic Change: Managing Cultural Processes," in Fahey and Randall, 1994, pp. 410–38.

4

The Approach to Strategic Plan Implementation

> When you change dramatically how the business is conducted,
> you transform the business itself.
>
> —*Stan Davis and Bill Davidson*

Executive Summary

The framework for effective strategic plan implementation is based on three principles:

1. *articulation:* using the organization's vision and values to align employees with its strategic direction
2. *activation:* completing the plan's action steps
3. *ability:* making sure employees have the skills to carry out the plan's new activities

Plan implementation is, in many ways, the most difficult step in the strategic planning process. Here, commitment to planning often faces its greatest challenges:

- executing the plan successfully
- ensuring that employees are sufficiently prepared for their roles in the plan's implementation
- managing the different timetables (plan development is a time-limited process, whereas implementation stretches over several years)
- determining how to acquire or develop the necessary capabilities for the strategic direction

INTRODUCTION

Once the strategic plan is completed and approved, it is ready for official implementation. The implementation process involves the organization's

111

entire employee base and affiliated organizations, as well as the medical staff. Although the number of participants involved in formulating and finalizing the strategic directions is relatively small, the scope of the project becomes enormous when the participation of those affected by its decisions is factored in. It is this dramatic shift that often determines the ultimate success or failure of the implementation.

This chapter presents a framework to approach effective strategic plan implementation that responds to or avoids commonly stated problems. It also discusses the problems and difficulties in plan implementation, including lack of organizational alignment, failure to measure expected and actual impact, and other problems related to transition. The following sections examine in detail the three principles of strategic plan implementation.

ARTICULATION

The engagement of employees in the plan's strategic direction should begin early, because leaders will strive for an organization-wide understanding of the environmental factors that drive the organization's vision, values, and strategic initiatives. Presenting this vital information in personal, nonthreatening situations provides employees the opportunity to offer input and feedback that may be useful in later implementation stages.

Employee involvement affects both the work design and reward systems. Employees' success or failure in implementing key initiatives can establish patterns for future workload assignments, and their participation in strategic teams can determine the scope of performance management systems that reward such participation. Employee involvement in acquiring expert knowledge in specific areas includes organization-provided training and education. The following systems, when incorporating strategic priorities, reinforce employee acceptance of the vision and value statements:

- performance reviews with measurable objectives, standards, and accomplishments
- general systems that provide management, human resources, and customer information support
- defined quality and service standards
- long- and short-range operations planning and annual budgeting
- human resources development and training
- formal and informal organizational structures (such as the team process)
- internal and external communications[1]

The meaning of the corporate vision and values will be enhanced if each division can identify the activities it takes part in to support the vision.

Benefits of such articulation include getting local support for the plan and hearing the kinds of questions and concerns that people may have about the corporate direction. In addition, articulation leads to the development of local service goals or standards that emulate the vision. Staff support is necessary for quality implementation and active participation in enhanced service delivery. In concert with the values statement, the staff's adaptation of the vision is an important part of conveying how the organization does business.

Finally, articulating the vision and progress toward set strategic directions comes from regular and constant discussion of the environment and the progress made toward the achievement of the vision. At middle management and departmental meetings, updates about progress toward the vision are essential to the continued involvement of the entire organization. Relying solely on internal, written communications from the communications department or senior management might encourage a perception, on the employees' part, of a barrier between them and the plan's initiators. If the employees view the plan as removed from their purposes and concerns and believe that they have neither input in the plan's development nor a stake in its success, the entire project could be jeopardized.

Organizations should take three steps to articulate their vision, values, and strategy:

1. Communicate the drivers for strategy direction.
2. Articulate the adaptation of the organization's vision and values.
3. Establish structures that support employee participation.

Communicate the Drivers for Strategy Direction

Discussing why the organization is revising its strategic direction sets a tone of openness about the shared problems and the shared responses to those problems. This process is also a necessary step in reinforcing the value and importance of the employees. It engages them in the same challenges that the board and senior management face and provides them with a context to better understand the direction of the organization. Such a discussion also gives employees some background to understand initiatives later undertaken to achieve the vision.

Organizations must assist their employees in expanding their understanding of the external environment. Such an understanding includes solid assessments of the competitors, the payers, the customers' requirements, and the choices and options available to the customers. The more comprehensive this understanding, the higher the employees' potential to take part in problem solving and to understand the context of resulting changes.

Informing the employee base in this way has additional benefits: It sets a context for any cost-cutting changes that may be required and enables management to announce any drastic changes internally, prior to their being reported in the media. The public attention currently surrounding the health care industry means that many organizational changes are broadcast by the press. Taking the initiative to communicate those to employees prior to the public announcement enhances the trust level.

Continuous internal updates about the implementation progress reinforce the message about strategic change with the physicians and employees. It also signals that management is committed to the shared vision and values, building a sense of interdependence. Even the updates on those initiatives that were explored but not undertaken, or failed initiatives, send an important message to employees, encouraging them to take risks and innovate at all levels of the organization.

Channels for Communicating the Completed Strategy Communication can occur via a variety of channels. While it is assumed that the strategy options have been tested with operational staff and physicians, further communication of the completed strategy may be more effective in smaller circles. Presentations can take place in small groups with middle managers and physicians. The greater the repetition, the greater the likelihood that employees will understand and integrate it.

A combination of channels can be helpful to repeat the vision and strategy. Annual meetings, quarterly or monthly meetings, formal meetings, informal meetings, and written communication, as well as all training programs, popularizes the vision and makes its relevance to the organization clear. The following is a list of possible media that health care organizations can use to communicate effectively with their employees:

- *Centralized presentations:* Used correctly, centralized presentations can be solid mechanisms for communicating strategic change. Such presentations, made in meetings with senior and middle managers, can keep leaders apprised of financial challenges and solicit their input in strategy development initiatives. A large forum is not always conducive to discussion and comments, however. Centralized presentations are most effective when used in conjunction with smaller follow-up meetings and other opportunities for two-way communication.
- *Internal newsletters and updates:* Internal communication media, such as the physician newsletter, the employee newsletter, and the employee magazine, are useful vehicles for updating the organization about key issues.
- *Departmental presentations:* Smaller, informal presentations that managers can use for their divisions and departments allow can-

did discussion about the direction of organization-wide changes and their relevance to each department.

- *E-mail from the president or CEO:* This is the fastest means of communication, and can be used to apprise physicians and employees about immediate changes or politically sensitive issues. E-mail can prevent physicians and employees from discovering new developments in their own organization from the press.

Organizations share strategic information in order to create a common framework for the employees and staff. Communication about the challenges and the overall direction of the organization reinforces the framework. Often, the method by which information is communicated has as much effect as the information itself. Figure 4-1 shows the results of one study involving the preferred methods of communication shared by physicians and administrators.

The impact of articulating strategic choices is powerful. In a commentary on the importance of presenting a strategy, Henry Mintzberg notes an example of how strong communication made the strategy more of a reality: "During the Vietnam conflict, when President Lyndon Johnson formally articulated the strategy of escalation that had been emerging over the previous four years, the bureaucracy ran with it far beyond his expectations—they overrealized the explicated strategy—and it subsequently became that much more difficult to stop. The more clearly the

FIGURE 4-1. Preferred Ways to Communicate between
               Management and Physicians

In a 1995 study, Premier noted the preferred ways to communicate between management and physicians (ranked here in order of importance):

Administrators' Preferred Methods of Communicating with Physicians

1. 1-on-1 meetings
2. Visits to physician services departments
3. Personal letter or call
4. Medical department meetings

Practicing Physicians' Preferred Methods of Communicating with Physicians

1. 1-on-1 meetings
2. M.D. advisory boards
3. Personal letter or phone calls from executives

Chief Medical Officers' Preferred Methods of Communicating with Physicians:

1. 1-on-1 meetings
2. Medical department meetings
3. Visits from physician services departments and personal letter/phone calls

Source: "Doctors Are from Mars, Hospital Execs from Venus" *Modern Healthcare* (Oct. 21, 1996): 79.

strategy is articulated, the more deeply embedded it becomes, in both the habits of the organization and the minds of its people. Thus the greater becomes its momentum."[2]

Example of Effective Communication   Experts emphasize the importance of keeping employees informed about the financial pressures facing the organization, the driving factors in the environment, and the progress of collaboration discussions. According to Laura Avakian, senior vice president of Care Group and Beth Israel Deaconess Medical Center, "Employees are told as much as the administration knows about our financial situation. Even 'bad news' is accepted better when employees are kept abreast of developments all the time instead of just being contacted when the crisis bell is tolling. If that happens," Avakian said, "year in and year out, there is a confidence that when you hear [news], it will be the truth.

"During affiliations discussions, the Beth Israel administrators make no secret of their (previous) ongoing talks with Lahey Hitchcock Clinic that could eventually result in organizational change at both institutions."[3]

Articulate the Adaptation of the Organization's Vision and Values

Individual divisions and departments may adapt the vision and values statement for their own puposes. When specific, localized objectives are tied to the vision and values statement, local support and understanding of the impact of the corporate strategy are much easier to obtain, and employees are able to anticipate opportunities to implement the strategy at an operational level. Dr. Richard Shea, vice president of medical affairs at Morton Plant Mease Health Care, illustrates how organizations must constantly incorporate vision and values in both job definition and required education:

> The job function is defined by the scope of responsibilities, which sets both the actual job duties and the impact of quality and service excellence goals. Individual and team performance are linked to the corporate strategy of quality and service excellence. Eight hours of quality awareness training are part of the orientation of all new employees to the health system, with 16- and 32-hour courses required for all members of management. The CEO is a regular participant in these educational sessions. At these and other regular meetings, the performance goals of individual work groups are regularly tied to achievement of a strategic direction, and progress with this process is reported on a quarterly basis to the Board of Directors.[4]

The emphasis on the vision and values statement directs changes in strategy and articulates the reasons for the changes that take place throughout the organization. This emphasis can align those who participate in the strategy and can provide gains in job satisfaction, energizing a large workforce to participate in change rather than be overwhelmed by it. As Henry Mintzberg points out: "Deep commitment, all-out support, is a necessary prerequisite to the successful pursuit of difficult courses of action. And that commitment seems to grow out of personal control, a sense of ownership of a project (hence the popularity of the word 'champion'), not deeply constrained by the specifics of form plans or the detachment of so-called objective calculations."[5]

Establish Structures That Support Employee Participation

Vision and strategy initiatives have implications for each of the organization's areas. With active participation in the implementation, the structure of work will inevitably change for some employees. For others, the changes in their work will be the result of the organization's transformation. These changed work activities can take the form of participation in strategic teams (discussed below) or in implementation of key initiatives. The changes, though, need to be defined and integrated into the performance management system.

Accomplishments may be recognized through such informal rewards as

- recognition
- control of resource allocation
- coveted assignments
- freedom from routine[6]

In addition, the organization must be willing to:

- *Permit the shifting of responsibilities to allow for time spent on strategic initiatives:* The time employees devote to strategic work should be factored into the composition of daily duties rather than assigned in addition to current duties. Other responsibilities may need to be shifted or postponed in order to ensure that quality work time is devoted to the team's direction. Although the participation of operational personnel is critical, shifting responsibilities may be more difficult for them than for those in staff functions. Ironically, if staff are able to absorb time-consuming projects on top of their current workload, it may appear that they have too much free time in their current roles.
- *Encourage systems support for employees:* In a further assessment of strategy implementation success factors, the requirement for systems support of employees is essential for employee alignment. As L. G. Hrebiniak and W. F. Joyce note, "Proper understanding of

motivation and appropriate use of incentives and controls are central to the successful implementation of strategy. Considerable time spent on the formulation of long-term objectives and elaborate plans for their achievement may, in fact, be wasted if incentives and controls result in behavior that is inconsistent with intended results."[7]

- *Reward strategic behavior with an established merit system:* The ability to function in a climate of change, whether toward further integration or resolution of operating problems that have plagued an organization, should be recognized. Those employees and staff members who have responsibility for the success of key initiatives also should be rewarded for enlisting those whose participation is needed to fulfill the vision.

These are the factors that reward different behaviors in a changing organization, as employees are asked to fulfill different duties with different accountability. These items will help to reward change and experimentation. Even more important than reinforcing participation is rewarding anticipatory thinking. Those who anticipate the change coming in their organization and act appropriately should be recognized.

Example of Performance Management Restructuring The importance of aligning individual performance with the strategic direction of the organization should be reflected in the organizational structure, the decision-making process in the management team, and finally in the way people are paid for their work. The following example of how one organization approached consolidation details deliberate steps that were taken to align the new organization with the way people are paid.

When Crozer-Keystone Health System consolidated four hospitals under two licenses in 1995, one management team ran the whole system, rather than four. Of that change, one executive noted, "When we started operating as a single team, people began to look at the whole picture. The territorial issues diminished quickly. The move made an enormous difference. There was also a change in the boards, so that the governing triumvirate was parent, health services, and health access."

In the process, Crozer-Keystone's leaders realized that they had created a reward system with internal incongruity; that is, the system's own financial reward structure worked against togetherness. Of that another executive remarked, "We had incentive plans in which an individual corporation could do exceedingly well, while the system went bankrupt. Even so, an individual would still be rewarded for how well he or she ran a corporation. We've changed that. Now rewards move across all corporations. The incentive is how well the system does. When the system downsized by 300 FTEs, few people had to go out the door. With every effort made to keep employees . . . the level of trust was higher than if the existing employees didn't have the commitment from management."[8]

Such a system calls for the coordination of the plan's implementation with designation of the accountable parties and proactive management of the update process. It signals a commitment from the management team to effectively schedule the implementation action plan in a timely fashion. In addition, such a system directs the attention of senior management to the implementation steps and balances the requirements of implementation with the daily requirements of running a business.

Establishment of Decentralized Work Groups To allow for flexibility and adaptation in establishing structures that support employee participation in strategic change, decentralized work groups can be created to pay particular attention to the impact on operations and business development. The team approach fosters an interdisciplinary process, which keeps the required functions attendant to both the operation and the new tactics as they are implemented.

These work teams will require a means to obtain customer feedback, in order to understand new environmental factors driving the strategy. This information gathering and dissemination must be part of the senior management review process and always shared with those who are part of the implementation.

ACTIVATION

Activation completes the strategic plan while allowing for a flexible process. Leaders must keep the plan's completion on the management's and the board's agendas and take strategic actions while keeping up with environmental and customer factors that call for revision. Described more fully in chapter 5, activation is discussed here as the concrete conceptualization of the initiatives as they are transformed from vision concepts into strategic directions.

Commitment from Management

Activation requires a commitment to manage action. Organizations must introduce change, whether by taking a strong company and making it stronger, or achieving a fast turnaround. An article on fast management turnaround notes five characteristics that apply to decisive leaders:

1. They show clear vision, charisma, and decisive leadership.
2. They change the old guard, the old culture—or both.
3. They tackle many problems at the same time.
4. They change how the companies' employees were judged and rewarded.
5. Their directors fully back their plans and hold them accountable.[9]

Leaders must create a balance between accepting and adjusting to change and moving forward with the implementation steps. Senior management, therefore, must pay attention to the implementation steps and balance the requirements of implementation with the daily requirements of running a business.

Requirements for Flexibility

The flexibility that organizations need to decentralize and revise their strategic direction requires the means to obtain customer feedback and understand new environmental factors that drive the strategy. The results of this information gathering and any indicated potential for modification of the strategy need to be shared with those who are part of the implementation work and who are responsible for its consequences.

As Theodore Levitt states, "Flexibility requires that organizations learn to move quickly. More than ever before, managerial effectiveness requires inspiration and shrewdness, fast decisions and firm decisiveness, courage linked to conviction, and above all, the will to act. It is becoming increasingly more important to act fast than to think correctly about tomorrow, because what one must act on is what is already in the process of happening, not what might happen later."[10]

Governance Oversight

Governance oversight is an ongoing function. Management's role in implementation consists of focusing on priorities and the completion of various steps in the process; analyzing the results; and proceeding to work on the subsequent strategy commitments. Oversight requires the designation of accountable individuals and the development of the support resources to conduct the implementation. The management review includes accounting for the initiatives being completed and working together to achieve results. The following example demonstrates how governance oversight affected the strategy implementation process in one organization.

A teaching hospital's leadership group composed of administrative managers, clinical chiefs, and the board's planning committee developed a strategic plan, which was approved by the board. The plan had a list of goal statements and support initiatives to be implemented by the management's strategic planning committee. The committee was made up of senior management and clinical chiefs, with the express purpose of maintaining the interests and issues of the medical school as part of the plan. Each action item was assigned to a member of the strategic planning committee for implementation, either directly or indirectly. Both the chair and co-chair were assigned, with the expectation that they would head a team of professionals who would assist with the work.

The strategic planning committee met quarterly and reviewed the reports from the team. Each chair and co-chair defined the scope of their work and its timeline. The oversight process was managed on a peer basis, and the progress was reported to the board.

The purpose of the senior management strategy discussions and update sessions is twofold: to manage the implementation process and to ensure completion of the goals and initiatives. This component of review and management has been deemed an essential part of strategy implementation. As H. I. Ansoff and R. C. Brandenburg note:

> Programming is a management activity that translates decisions into specific action patterns for implementation. The primary management tasks in this phase are:
> 1. scheduling activities in support of decision
> 2. assigning and scheduling of resources in support of decision (commonly referred to as budgeting)
> 3. establishing patterns of work flows in the firm
> 4. establishing patterns of authority and responsibility
> 5. establishing communication flow networks[11]

The flexibility of the plan relies upon a continual update on relevant factors in the environment and customer feedback. Monitoring of critical issues and environmental factors is continuous. Customer needs must be constantly assessed to ensure that the strategy is not based on outmoded customer assessments and the "seller's" idea of what needs to happen.

Activation of the Plan

Translating the plan into concrete directions and actions requires the creation of teams or task forces. The following subsections address some of the important factors organizations should consider when forming and implementing their teams.

Creation of Teams Teams can be composed of people who will either do the actual work or live with the impact of the outcome. In the first case, a working team will be responsible for all or most of the work. In the latter case, the team may be the customers or beneficiaries of a change. As part of the team's creation, its leaders should note the goals, the scope of work, the life of the team, and how much authority the team members have before requiring the approval of others. The process and ground rules by which a team does its work should be clarified.

Teams as Tools for Employee Alignment Teams can engage employees, offer reality tests during the development stage, and foster innovation throughout the organization. In addition to the formal mechanisms noted in chapter 5, the team approach also translates the conceptual initiatives in the broad vision statement to the concrete objectives. Finally, it sends the message of the importance of taking responsibility for and ownership of the vision throughout the organization.

Some organizations are taking a new, innovative tack. They use teams to develop products or concepts in ways that involve people close to the service delivery and to gain employee commitment to the overall direction. The employees' alignment is partly solved by the creation of teams, especially when they include the direct involvement of more junior staff. Using teams to resolve issues and problems improves the delivery of services at the operational level and encourages those outside senior management to commit to the strategic intent. Learning to work together as a team is one of the tools necessary to solve problems throughout the organization.

Diversity within Teams Forming teams made up of members from different areas and levels of the organization serves two purposes. First, organizations become more democratic. Second, people closer to the operations can take advantage of the "white space" opportunities—new areas of growth possibilities that fall between the cracks because they do not naturally match the skills of existing business units.

Because most health care initiatives interface with multiple functional areas, a "strategic team" can bring together staff who represent areas critical to the initiative's success. Formal planning literature also suggests that moving from strategy to implementation may falter due to lack of information and participation by those whose job it is to make an initiative succeed.

Examples of Successful Teams The successful use of teams has addressed many operational and strategy challenges, as shown by the following examples:

- At Allina Health System in Minneapolis, teams are used to address system snags and work through process problems and quality issues, staying active for as long as it takes to get the job done.

- Presbyterian Hospital in Dallas uses teams to complement patient-focused care and expects to save as much as $4.5 million by the end of 1997. The hospital has worked in teams for almost 6 years. Its 3,000 employees are organized into more than 30 teams. Presbyterian has documented increases in patient and staff satisfaction based on team implementation.[12]

ABILITY

Building ability sets into an organization's strategic planning ensures that employees have the proper skills and experience to implement strategy. Acute care hospitals are changing their service delivery, merging, and forming new alliances, and these new lines of business require new talents. Organizations have two options: (1) retraining their traditional acute care hospital employees in a broader range of service delivery and management or (2) acquiring new talent. Talents traditionally associated with related businesses and the ability to work well in the new paradigm of team learning are becoming increasingly critical attributes for health care employees. While some new capabilities can be taught, others require new staff or new affiliations with expert organizations to acquire those capabilities.

Where a need for retraining exists, the organization must commit to internal or external training. The scope of this retraining depends on the organization's structure and the level of change dictated by the new strategic direction.

The acquisition of expert knowledge, whether clinical or administrative, is sometimes necessary to ensure that the organization is not reinventing the wheel in its attempts to restructure itself from the ground up. This expert knowledge may involve an internal operating systems review by a technical expert and a review of other available operating systems to enhance or develop capabilities to support the initiative.

The commitment to change involves changes in service delivery, service definition, and the use of technology, both clinical and information. Some tasks the organization should undertake as part of the process of addressing required skills are listed below:

- Identify the skills needed to pursue the strategic vision
- Identify the competencies needed, in terms of both technical competence and process competence
- Identify the resources required to train existing staff
- Identify the areas in which new capabilities will be needed

As hospital-focused organizations evolve into health care systems that include physician practices and payer products, new priorities and skills are needed. The management of physician interests and practices, the management of subacute services, and the management of payer systems are markedly different from the skills associated with management in the hospital setting. The need for new types of management capabilities may be met by adaptable current staff or may call for new staff with expertise outside the hospital setting. With this change comes a fundamental shift in both clinical priorities and management focus, which requires new levels of competence for success.

Staff Training

As the inpatient care focus evolves into a provider focus, the technical competence required to manage a range of services must expand to include different clinical and business capabilities. Staff who can recognize opportunities and can respond independently make an enormous difference in an organization in the process of transformation. A practical application of this principle is illustrated in the following example.

Staff Training Case Example   New York Downtown Hospital is a 220-bed hospital with 1,000 employees. In 1991 the new CEO and management team decided that the professional development of the middle managers was critical to the hospital's successful adaptation, survival, and growth in a difficult and constantly changing health care market. The program that was created to answer this need consisted of formal training in the organization, with courses, projects, and assigned mentors. Senior managers who were designated mentors formalized this role, meeting to review their duties and program objectives. The mentors then nominated middle manager candidates, with 40 managers participating in the first year. Those selected for the program lacked formal management training or management experience prior to assuming their present positions. Mentors were assigned to middle managers who did not report to them and established learning contracts. The curriculum consisted of the following seminars in the first quarter:

1. customer services
2. financial management for nonfinancial managers
3. managing more effectively

Later seminar topics included continuous quality improvement, methods of staff motivation, leadership, communication, conflict management, managing cultural diversity, hiring and managing staff, and managing change. Some participants developed projects based on learning contract objectives, making the program a process of both classroom and experiential learning.

The program was supported by grant funds dedicated to developing new skills and capabilities in middle managers. At the conclusion of the first year, the following recommendations were developed to further enhance the program:

1. Continue the program after the grant.
2. Revise the program before the end of year two.
3. Develop guidelines for the expectations of mentors, participants, and supervisors.
4. Fund it internally.
5. Develop new and separate programs for physician executives holding management positions.
6. Make the program voluntary.[13]

Other Types of Staff Training In addition to leadership skills training, training about work style, information-processing preferences, and their implications for working together can generate appreciation for style synergies rather than resentment of dissimilarities. In this way, idea development, conflict, and the resolve to carry out ideas can be processed without personality dispute, and with a focus on innovation. Such training also lays the groundwork for the way team members deal with conflict and respond to the ideas of others. This approach can make the difference between responding with suspicion and responding with enthusiasm over a potential improvement in result or process.

Outside experts can often aid in the process of learning how to reach agreement. The transition from a nonteam to a team approach often requires technical assistance, such as conflict resolution or interactive listening skills.

Skill-specific training can be useful as an adjunct to team skill and management training. For example, customer service is a distinct competence. In a market where prices are similar, people make decisions based on their relationships with physicians. Better communication improves patient care, satisfaction, and compliance. One common challenge for health care providers is finding an inoffensive way of discussing financial issues with a patient without compromising the quality of care delivered. One health care organization that undertook a training initiative to prepare care providers for the challenges of customer service is Wayne State University Medical School in Detroit. With the funding of a partnership led by General Motors and dedicated to teaching physicians how to factor costs into treatment decisions, Wayne State University Medical School and a coalition of six hospitals will launch a training program for 10,000 doctors in southeastern Michigan. The partnership has pinpointed six areas of care where money can be saved if doctors are better trained concerning the results of their treatment decisions. These areas are

- prescription drug costs
- medical and surgical supplies and equipment

- diagnostic procedures
- durable medical equipment
- rehabilitation services
- workers' compensation services[14]

This initiative demonstrates how health care organizations are seeking ways to improve the delivery and cost of care by updating the internal environment and retraining their staff.

Team Training

Team training fosters the development of new business skills and the capabilities required to effect strategic transformation. The use of teams to implement changes in direction requires the leadership of a number of individuals who already possess outstanding team management and group development skills. Technical knowledge and team competence rarely coexist. No matter how talented the members of the team are as individuals, their success as a team depends on their competence at teamwork. Deploying talented team players strategically within developing teams can often return results greater than those created by selecting only the most technically competent.

The Saturn Corporation is a good example of positive trends in employee education and team development. Saturn was launched by parent company General Motors in order to build an American car that could compete with Japanese imports. To do so, executives realized that Saturn required both a technologically advanced environment and a highly skilled and motivated workforce. As a result, each employee, both management and union, spends over one hundred hours in training every year. This training process is described by Stan Davis in his book, *The Monster under the Bed:*

> Saturn employees start their formal training on "Excel," an experiential course. First, they go through a "blind trust walk" where one person is blindfolded and led by a teammate through an obstacle course. Second, they climb a forty-foot-high wall working together in teams of three. Third, they return to a class setting to discuss issues of truth, accountability, support, trust and empowerment. A set of individual and corporate values develops from these experiences, including a dedication to teamwork, a commitment to excel, trust and respect for the individual, acknowledgment of the necessity for continuous improvement, and commitment to build customer enthusiasm.[15]

Finally, it should be noted that the structure of discussion may be used to deal with complex team issues on a systemic basis. These discussions should focus on practical issues: "Without a shared language for dealing with complexity, team learning is limited. . . . There is simply no more effective way to learn a language than through use, which is exactly what happens when a team starts to learn the language of systems thinking."[16]

Skill Acquisition through Outsourcing

As noted previously, an organization can acquire the skills needed to perform new functions through training, hiring new talent, or forming alliances with experienced organizations. There are a range of partnership options: contract management, outsourcing, co-sourcing, and joint ventures. Contract management has long been an essential part of many health care organizations, for a variety of reasons. It is a means both of saving money and benefiting from the expertise of companies that focus on specific services. Outsourcing a function is becoming increasingly attractive in a range of different service fields. As the following example demonstrates, the resulting partnership allows the provider organization to acquire expert capabilities that deliver required services.

When Crozer-Keystone Health System determined that its strategy relied on information technology, it targeted several important initiatives:

- establishment of patient-centered data collection with timely reminders and customized informative letters through a complex database marketing application
- development of a longitudinal clinical record to streamline health management for patients and physicians
- construction of a facility to provide acute care, wellness, fitness, early intervention, and prevention programs to improve community health

Crozer-Keystone invested heavily in information technology to make the management of these programs possible, but soon realized that the ideas required more expertise than they had in house at the time, so they outsourced the information technology function to SMS. SMS is paid based on the fulfillment of rigorous performance service standards.[17]

Outsourcing decreases costs, saves on the development of specialized capabilities, and allows attention to be directed to other competency enhancement projects. Outsourcing is a common management activity, but must be viewed as more than a tactical tool. Long-term partnerships based on the fulfillment of performance standards are the mechanisms that mark successful outsourcing relationships for business and clinical services.

Finding expertise in key areas can also come from joint ventures. Partnerships create opportunities to move quickly into new areas and take advantage of core competencies of other organizations. Across all industries, forming partnerships is seen as a mechanism to acquire key competencies without having to take the time to develop the competence independently. The *Wall Street Journal* has reported, "Over half of America's fastest-growing companies have teamed with others during the past three years to improve products or create new ones."[18]

PAST PROBLEMS WITH STRATEGIC PLAN IMPLEMENTATION

Recent business literature tends to focus more on the problems organizations face during the implementation stage of their strategic plans than on their successes. Strategy literature generally identifies three such problems:

- measuring impact
- aligning the organization
- translating strategy into action

Responding to these factors will decrease the likelihood of strategy implementation failure. The following subsections discuss these problems in some detail, and offer some solutions for how organizations can circumvent them. Figure 4-2 lists some common errors in implementation.

Measuring Impact

There are those who resist the formality of the planning activity, arguing that it is no more effective than relying on the professional capabilities of

FIGURE 4-2. Failed Transformations Exhibit Plans, but No Vision

The following is a list of the most common errors organizations make when they attempt to implement a change in strategic direction.

Error 1: Not establishing a great enough sense of urgency

Error 2: Not creating a powerful enough guiding coalition

Error 3: Lacking a vision

Error 4: Under-communicating the vision by a factor of ten

Error 5: Not removing obstacles to the new vision

Error 6: Not systematically planning for and creating short term wins

Error 7: Declaring victory too soon

Error 8: Not anchoring changes in the corporation's culture

John Kotter, "Leading Change: Why Transformation Efforts Fail" *Harvard Business Review* (Mar.-Apr. 1995).

management without a framework of a planning effort. Because so many strategic planning endeavors have failed without objective study, it is difficult to involve the critics in a thoughtful review of the reasons for the failure.

One of the problems associated with evaluating the results of the strategic planning revolves around issues of measurement. As Henry Mintzberg notes, "A positive correlation between planning and performance allows no one to conclude that planning pays. Causation may also go the other way: only rich organizations can afford planning or at least planners . . . firms that do well naturally emphasize their planning activities (since they made or exceeded their targets) while those that do poorly become unsure of them and so underemphasize them . . . extensive measurement problems suggest that these findings underestimate the true relationship between planning and performance."[19])

The planning process should produce results that are measurable through tactics that contribute to the strategic directions. This connection is made with specific measures identified in the planning process. Without interrelated measurement systems—a way to systematically understand progress from one period to another—only intuition can establish a relationship between the planning process and its outcomes.

Two elements establish performance measurement systems for the strategic planning process:

- *Deciding what to measure:* Beyond the traditional financial measures that are outgrowths of centralized, controlled environments, measurements should include customer satisfaction, employee satisfaction, and productivity. Such information enables an organization to adjust more easily to changing external environments. The specific measures will vary among organizations, although the introduction of quality indicators creates a baseline set of data. Consistency in measurement over time is almost as important as the specific elements chosen to measure. Even with defining success criteria, it is difficult to gauge success in a rapidly changing environment. Therefore, while a strategic plan may be implemented over a period of years, the annual review and criteria for success should be updated based on completed goals.
- *Establishing systems to achieve consistency:* Systems can be put in place to capture and report outcomes of strategic initiatives. Organizations require advanced information technology, committed leadership, and thorough analysis to understand the results of performance measurement systems. The capture of data and their presentation must have a consistency across measurement periods that fosters such thoughtful analysis.

Measurement systems require time and input from the employees and staff that provide and use the information. Those organizations that have been most successful with this approach have expended substantial resources over an extended period of time. But the value of such decision-making information can be seen in the level of success of those organizations that have made such commitments.

Aligning the Organization

Organizational alignment is more than the process of letting people know about the direction of the organization. It is continual interaction that invokes the active voluntary participation of the employees, the supporters, and the volunteers of the organization in creating the future of the organization as expressed in the vision. The alignment of these people is necessary to achieve the strategic outcomes and make significant changes to achieve the vision.

Guiding Employees through Change   Articulating the vision and values is essential to guiding employees through change. The focus on the development of a vision manifests itself in the formal and informal processes that ensure employee commitment to participating in the organization's future. These processes communicate the structure of the organization and the technical components of its performance. Such parts include reward systems for achieving objectives and the training and talent acquisition that will make the changes possible.

The change in process and organizational culture necessarily includes a new approach to both innovation and teamwork. Implementation may call for dramatic changes. A change as profound as a paradigm shift (from a focus on a high volume of acute care encounters to a focus on high volume of covered lives with greatest care efficiency) requires changes in care delivery and resource allocation. It also requires different incentives for different types of behaviors and successes. Each employee must be able to visualize his or her own role and its importance in attaining the vision.

Finding New Leaders   New kinds of problem solving and teamwork require new skills and considerations about other colleagues. This shift has to be reinforced by new approaches to performance management, leadership actions, values statement articulation and dissemination, and each department's specific goals.

Such management techniques include involving employees and constituents in planning the future of the organization and in translating the vision into actions. Therefore, employees need role models, leaders whose actions reflect the intended new directions. Without leaders who reflect the strategic vision in their own work and communications, employees may lack confidence in their stated directions.

One community health care organization developed a decentralized approach to product line management and development. Each product line leader is expected to produce a business plan to develop or improve his or her specific service, and a team is responsible for the work. The time frame allows months for the development of the business plans, at the end of which the CEO reviews and approves them. Those plans not approved are left until next year's cycle.

For those initiatives that were approved, the work teams' results were rewarded with recognition. But for those work teams whose initiatives that were not approved were unable to proceed. The ensuing business plan development was not managed with enthusiasm. Thus, the importance of the stated direction of the organization becomes lost without an overall sense of direction provided by an articulated, organization-wide vision.

Getting Employees Invested In short, lost opportunities often have to do with failing to invigorate the employees and to get them invested in the overall direction of the organization. The temptation to motivate by highlighting successes can result in the perception that the required work has been done. While noting successes along the way is important to achieving change, real success will come with the movement toward operationalizing the vision. Rewards are important, but the way business is conducted must reflect the vision: How communication takes place and how improved processes are introduced reinforce the values needed for success. The mission statement reflects the business of the organization, and the old strategic plan reflects actions to be taken; the vision, however, portrays the future picture, and the values dictate what actions will help to reach that future.

Translating Strategy into Action

Once an organization has made a commitment to a strategic approach or plan, the leadership, management team, and employees and staff must move to implement the plan. The activation of the vision and values statement articulates the future of the organization and allows flexibility in the implementation process. The driving force in the implementation is to achieve the vision in concert with the values. Two particular problems must be addressed in order to achieve effective implementation: (1) insufficient freedom to gain buy-in and (2) lack of reality testing.

Insufficient Freedom to Gain Buy-in The plan has to be able to conform to operations rather than exist as a separate organism developed by a planning team and senior management. Operations staff function differently than the people around the planning table. In many organizations, implementation has been plagued by the problems of having insufficient freedom to gain buy-in for the plan and having too many constraints on the implementation. As Henry Mintzberg states, "Each implementor must inevitably retain some discretion, to interpret intended strategies in his or her own way."[20]

Health care organizations have been faulted for overanalyzing business opportunities prior to taking action, leading to a cycle called "analysis paralysis"—when analysis takes the place of rapid response to the environment. Because of the long-standing luxury of cost-based reimbursement, health care organizations have not had to go beyond predicting their own payment changes.

Many analysts agree that strategy is often lost during implementation. That may be due in part to the separation between those who plan and those who implement. There is a critical need for communication and buy-in between these parties, for "strategic intentions get distorted or deflected on their way to implementation."[21]

Lack of Reality Testing Another failure in strategy implementation is the lack of reality testing. The lack of sufficient reality testing with the people or systems that will be most affected by the initiative often means that important aspects are overlooked. The people who develop the initiatives may be too removed from the implementation and, in their haste to implement an initiative, might miss the chance to formulate parameters that mirror the shared vision for that business.

Failure to manage the strategy and vision implementation in the organization results in a failure to enlist employees and physicians in the strategic direction. If a health care system holds the public relations department alone accountable for the employee awareness and understanding of the vision and strategy, the opportunity to state and restate the vision and strategy is limited. (Operational staff also should be involved in disseminating information.) With a limited understanding of the vision and strategic direction, there may be a drift in the understanding and integration of strategy into the organization.

CONCLUSION

Effective strategic plan implementation is based on three principles: articulation, activation, and ability. The organization that can successfully impart the new direction to employees, complete its plan's action steps, and make sure that employees have the skills to carry out new activities must avoid the pitfalls of implementation, which are some of the most challenging of the entire strategic planning process.

References

1. B. B. Tregoe, and others, *Vision in Action: Putting a Winning Strategy to Work* (New York: Simon and Schuster, 1989), p. 119.

2. Henry Mintzberg, *The Rise and Fall of Strategic Planning* (New York: The Free Press, 1994), p. 175.

3. "Hospital Administrators Try to Keep up Morale Even as They Cut Staff," *Boston Business Journal* 15 (Aug. 1995): 8-9.

4. Interview with Dr. Richard Shea, vice president of medical affairs at Morton Plant Mease Health Care, 1996.

5. Henry Mintzberg, *The Rise and Fall of Strategic Planning*, p. 172.

6. Warren Bennis and Burt Nanus, *Leaders: The Strategies for Taking Charge* (New York: HarperPerennial, 1988), p. 206.

7. L. G. Hrebiniak and W. F. Joyce, *Implementing Strategy* (New York: Macmillan, 1984), p. 213.

8. "Tiptoeing toward Nirvana," *Hospitals and Heath Networks Pacesetters* (Nov. 1996): 12-13.

9. "How Three CEOs Achieved Fast Turnarounds," *Wall Street Journal* (Spring 1995): b1.

10. Theodore Levitt, *Thinking About Management* (New York: The Free Press, 1991), p. 95.

11. H. I. Ansoff and R. C. Brandenburg, "A Program of Research in Business Planning," *Management Science* XIII, no. 6 (1967):B225-B226.

12. Chuck Appleby, "Betting against Health Care," *Hospitals & Health Networks* 70 (July 5, 1996): 34.

13. Anthony Kovner and others, "Management Development for Mid-Level Managers: Results of a Demonstration Project," *Hospital and Health Services Administration* 41, no. 4 (1996): 485-502.

14. *Modern Healthcare* 26 (Jan. 13, 1996): 17.

15. Stan Davis, *The Monster Under the Bed* (New York: Simon and Schuster, 1994), pp. 86-87.

16. *Wall Street Journal* (Jan. 9, 1997): 1.

17. "Chunk of Change," Hospitals and Health Networks Pacesetters (Nov. 1996): 16-21.

18. *Wall Street Journal* (Jan. 9, 1997).

19. Henry Mintzberg, *The Rise and Fall of Strategic Planning*, pp. 92-97.

20. Ibid., p. 286.

21. Ibid., p. 286.

5

Action Steps in Strategic Plan Implementation

Without a gardener, there's no garden.

—*Stephen Covey*

Executive Summary

One of the greatest challenges in implementing a strategy is aligning employees in new directions. Developing vision and values statements are the first steps in aligning employees, and the subsequent articulation of these statements is critical in making the alignment work. Successful strategic implementation also requires ensuring that employees have the necessary abilities and training to realize the new directions.

To help develop a sense of accountability in the organization for accomplishing the initiatives, members of the senior management team oversee an initiative and use an interdisciplinary team or task force approach to implement the initiative.

INTRODUCTION

The implementation process starts as soon as the strategic plan is approved or, in highly sensitive situations requiring prompt action, before the plan is completed. A review process is needed for coordinating efforts and addressing issues that arise during implementation.

Successful implementation is a team effort, requiring accountability and flexibility. The organization must adopt a flexible approach to inculcating the entire employee base and acquiring necessary talent from outside the organization.

Involving staff from all levels of an organization—an increasingly "democratic" process—is essential. Such democratization, nevertheless, places responsibility on management, because accountability, focused attention on the efforts, and thorough process reporting are all required in the successful implementation of a strategic plan.

This chapter reviews the components of implementation, discussing activities necessary to achieve the vision and incorporate the organizational values. It provides examples of some progressive means of integrating, responding to, and preparing for greater levels of managed care, as well as developing new approaches to collaborative marketing. Contingencies and the resolution of new challenges found during implementation are also discussed.

COMPONENTS OF THE IMPLEMENTATION PROCESS

Implementation includes the following processes:

- designating accountability for the initiatives
- focusing management attention on the implementation
- reporting on implementation progress
- moving the organization toward change
- rewarding change and experimentation

The following subsections discuss these components in detail.

Designating Accountability

Being "accountable" for an initiative means taking responsibility for achieving the desired outcome. The first step is for management to review the action plan and assign accountability for the initiatives. The planning process will result in a list of directions and anticipated actions for the organization, to be implemented over a multiyear period, with suggested time frames. This list is then translated into a project list, designating responsible persons to lead each project and proposing timetables for completion. That may be accomplished by a combined work task force, with a senior manager leading the process internally or engaging and managing outside talent to complete an initiative.

Make Someone Accountable There are several models for designating accountability. One model involves designating an accountable senior manager. Another involves making the developers of the strategy responsible for the strategy's implementation. Another model is to develop a central team authority. However, this method often suffers from the lack of one person as a driving force.

Another model is that of shared leadership of an initiative. The commitment to implementation is achieved by assigning plan participants responsibility for the outcomes. When action plans are managed by a group of peers, an often frustrating sense of hierarchy during the implementation and review process is avoided.

Obtain Top-Level Management Support Top-level management support is essential for the success of any initiative. One way to signal that this support is present is to have one senior manager, if not direct management, charged with overseeing the initiative. Specific senior management meetings can be scheduled on a regular basis to review the strategic implementation progress. As the planning committee meets, it may also be advised of the implementation progress.

Define the Reporting Structure Once a responsible senior manager or team of senior managers is assigned responsibility for each initiative, then regular meetings should be scheduled, at which strategy progress will be monitored. The senior management team, or a similarly composed physician council (assuming there is physician participation) thereby takes responsibility for the initiatives. Results of these meetings may be shared among members of the planning committee and then also shared with the board. The employees and affiliated partners should also be updated regularly. Following the maxim "Go public and go often" is an important part of implementation success.

Define the Terms of Accountability In order to achieve completion of the strategic initiatives, management must make the terms for accountability clear. Moreover, an incentive system for the meaningful completion of the initiatives must also be made clear. Finally, the leaders of the initiatives must implement a definitive reporting structure. There are two ways to accomplish these goals:

1. Make the process of realizing strategic change part of the standing merit performance system and part of the annual performance review. Change, such as toward further consolidation or toward resolving operating problems that have plagued the organization, necessitates aligning the players. Those who have responsibility for the success of key initiatives have to be rewarded both for inculcating those whose participation is needed as well as for their contribution to the fulfillment of the vision.

2. Make the process of realizing strategic change part of the organization's culture and values. Successful implementation requires

top management to actively and visibly support innovation and creative thinking; thoughtful risk-taking, even in cases of ultimate failure, should be encouraged rather than reproached.

Focusing Management Attention

It is important to bring progress in implementation to both the formal and informal attention of the management team. Informally, communications and the articulation of the strategic initiatives have to take place, particularly as work processes and activities are redesigned. Ongoing formal attention occurs as part of the regular strategy update sessions.

Purpose of Senior Management Strategy Meetings The purpose of the senior management strategy discussion and update sessions is to review and manage the implementation, thereby ensuring completion of the goals and initiatives. This component of review has been deemed an essential part of strategy implementation and can be traced to planning literature of at least 30 years ago, as the following attests:

> Programming is a management activity that translates decisions into specific action patterns for implementation. The primary management tasks in this phase are:
> - scheduling activities in support of decision
> - assignment and scheduling of resources in support of decision (commonly referred to as budgeting)
> - establishing patterns of work flows in the firm
> - establishing patterns of authority and responsibility
> - establishing communication flow networks[1]

Focused, regular attention to the implementation of the strategic plan on the part of the organization's senior management, including the CEO, will allow for smoother progress. It decreases the possibility of surprise, provides early recognition of problems, and allows for flexibility in changing a strategy that is not working. Moreover, regular attention and feedback inspires employees to continue with their efforts.

The discussion of activation in chapter 4 reviewed the process one tertiary hospital management team adopted in assigning accountability for strategy implementation. In this scenario, the management team consisted of both senior administrators and clinical chiefs, a team structure that ensured that medical staff leadership was participating in initiatives and was regularly updated on new developments. Similarly, strategy updates provide management with an opportunity to understand fully the impact of new processes on other departments.

When the review and control process is overseen by a senior management team, the plan becomes an active part of the organization in the following six ways:

- by measuring the continued relevance of the issues identified in the plan
- by evaluating the analytical framework of the strategy and tactics
- by developing course correction if or as needed
- by reviewing the plan with changed leadership in the board, medical staff, and management
- by modifying service delivery (closing/expansion/development) plans based on performance of key variables
- by providing early recognition of issues

Structure and Agenda of the Strategy Meetings The management team might choose to schedule strategy meetings on a regular basis—separate from regular management meetings—in order to focus on the strategic agenda and review the tactical plan. These meetings may be several hours in length, depending on their frequency and the depth of the discussion. The agenda for such meetings might read as follows:

- strategic updates (new events or data relevant to the organization's direction)
- project status for projects in progress this year
- status of infrastructure preparation
- fiscal services (operating budget)
- marketing
- information systems
- human resources
- facilities

This agenda allows discussion and review of the projects as well as new issues affecting the projects. New information may require the plan's revision; such variables underscore the importance of allocating enough discussion time.

A meeting among senior staff should be held on a monthly basis to review the projects due that quarter and discuss projects in progress. The meeting may include discussion of timing and deadlines, impact on current operations, and any updates on the project. For each project, initiative, or action item, the following elements should be noted:

- goal
- objective/initiative
- tactic/project
- lead person

- start date
- completion date
- resources
- monitoring measures
- status

Using the above information, projects can be organized by category, lead person, or start and completion dates. Capturing information in this fashion can also allow for comparisons with other initiatives.

In a recent management magazine, interviews with strategists whose work has become increasingly important in the business sector emphasized staff involvement:

> Today's gurus of strategy urge companies to democratize the process—once the sole province of a company's most senior officers—by handing strategic planning over to teams of line and staff managers from different disciplines. Frequently, these teams include junior staffers, hand-picked for their ability to think creatively, and near-retirement old-timers willing to tell it like it is. . . . To keep the planning process close to the realities of markets today, strategists should also include interaction with key customers and suppliers. That openness alone marks a revolution in strategic planning, which was always among the most sacrosanct and clandestine of corporate activities. But it's necessary if the process is to help produce what customers want.[2]

It is important to note, however, that even in a democratic process such as that described above, the organization retains the right to choose how and when to involve employees and when to begin delegating key initiative developments and refinements.

Reporting on Implementation Progress

The updates on the progress of the strategy implementation should consider items accomplished as well as those yet to be addressed. Moreover, they may include reports on the expected impact of the completed actions or new issues that may arise from completion. The impact of completed initiatives should be considered in terms of their actual and expected effect on the organization's bottom line. In the event of a volume or financial consequence, the monitoring of that expected outcome should commence immediately. If expected outcomes cannot be monitored in terms of volume or financial consequences, management needs to develop an alternative system of measurement.

The review and reporting process facilitates the plan's implementation schedule. Ongoing attention to the action plan ensures that the plan will not rest on a shelf unused.

Groups to Which Progress Should Be Reported Progress reports on the implementation of the strategic plan should be made regularly available to the leadership groups: middle management, the medical staff, and the board. Whether this is a part of standard monthly or quarterly group meetings or is addressed at special update sessions, the organization's progress in strategic directions needs continuing attention.

Presentation of the updates on strategy implementation, in terms of areas actively undertaken and those found not feasible, sends an important message to employees that innovation and risk-taking are underway at all levels of the organization. Bringing special attention to, rather than downplaying, those efforts that were tried and failed shows the value the organization places on innovation.

Updates on the accomplishments of strategically important initiatives should also be shared with new employee groups. Some organizations use newsletter updates effectively for this purpose. Employee communications and activities should be shared with people from new areas or divisions, so that a sense of interdependence builds. That also aids in integrating employees into strategically relevant parts of the organization.

Reports to the Overseeing Committee The committee that oversees the plan—whether a planning committee or the executive committee—also needs to be updated about the progress of the strategic implementation. Such reports should be made regularly and may restate prior plan expectations for purposes of comparison. While management is accountable for the implementation of the strategic plan, the guidance of the leadership group in strategic plan matters is as important as their overseeing the finances of the organization.

Reports to the Board The progress on the strategic initiatives and the expected next steps should be shared with the board. If expected outcomes are monitored in terms of volume and financial reports, changes should be noted in the regular reporting structure. The report to the board can be made through the planning committee report or, again, included as part of the CEO's report. The medical staff update can be made either as a medical executive committee presentation or included as part of the CEO's report.

The board assures the success of the health care organization in terms of both its financial management and its orientation to its mission and service intent. For a hospital, this role has been defined by Mary K. Totten as tuned "to the needs of the community and with keeping the hospital true to its mission. Yet it is also the trustee who must make certain that the hospital is able to respond to changes in the environment and survive for the long term to continue to provide its much-needed services."[3] The board's interest in the implementation of the strategic plan, of which some members will have a significant role in development, is likely to be more than just passing.

As the board reviews the plan's implementation, there may be modifications of the original plan, such as the following:

- Rearrange the expected timetable of particular projects.
- Reallocate resources to explore and resolve projects.
- Reprioritize projects and the timetable.
- Initiate projects that meet strategic direction but were not on the initial list.

Moving the Organization toward Change

Changing an organization's direction and asking staff to be part of this change requires innovative tactics. The five components relevant to achieving a vision, according to Peter Senge in *The Fifth Discipline,* are discussed below.

1. *Systems thinking:* This concept of health care delivery is broader than the acute care model and encompasses care starting with primary care physicians services (augmented by specialists), subacute and home care services, and acute care services.
2. *Personal mastery:* The process of personal mastery involves how employees personally revise and clarify their own role in health care delivery. With the change in the health care organization and change in the focus of care for the patient, employee roles will likely change and new roles will need mastering. While such "personal mastery" is more fully explored in the "ability" section of chapter 4, it here serves as an essential step in meeting new organizational challenges.
3. *Mental models:* Building mental models is a means of challenging assumptions about every part of the health care delivery system. New "mental models" take into consideration quantitative data, other conceptual models, and finally the vision for the health care organization. The delivery system—individuals, work groups, departments, and divisions—will need to be redrawn as the health care organization and industry evolves.
4. *Building shared vision:* This process is a means of acknowledging, enacting, and celebrating the future of the organization. The shared commitment of the employees and management to the organization's future is necessary for realizing the plan-developed vision.
5. *Team learning:* This activity uses the input of employees who are close to operations, rather than that of higher management, in rewriting the nuances of a specific service delivery. The process that teams engage in when they think together is necessary for problem solving and inventing new modes of delivery.[4]

Rewarding Change and Experimentation

During the articulation of the vision and strategic directions, there are a variety of ways to encourage a work force to operate in a different way. The performance management systems that reward new behaviors are both formal and informal. They include

- compensation
- recognition
- allowing control over resource allocation
- formal promotion
- making special assignments
- allowing latitude in expense accounts
- providing freedom and flexibility from routine constraints[5]

As rewards for employees who are asked to do different work with different accountability, these items will help to encourage change and experimentation. Perhaps even more important than reinforcing participation is rewarding anticipatory thinking; those who anticipate change and act early to adapt should be recognized.

In addition to formal training and skill development, employees are encouraged to adopt new behaviors through the retooling of performance reviews to reward a "new" or newly articulated set of values. Organizations must be able to continue motivating employees in this fashion to align them in strategic endeavors.

MOVING TOWARD MANAGED CARE AND INTEGRATION

The anticipation of widespread payer-required capitation, and the ensuing interest in capitation and global payments, emphasizes the integrated delivery system (IDS) as a significant, industry-wide strategic direction. An organization's strategic intent is identified in both its vision and, more specifically, in its action plan. Many action plans in more recent years have placed increasing emphasis on IDSs and capitation. Many marketplaces differ in terms of interest in capitation. The opportunity for choice among providers is of interest to most consumers, but it is uncertain whether more integration will provide more choices. In any case, making deliberate decisions about approaching capitation for real expected outcomes has to be actively managed.

Continuing to focus on movement toward more managed care will play an increasingly important role through the 1990s in holding down costs for payers. Success in this arena relies on managing the following areas:

- payer involvement
- physician network development
- organizational and financial capabilities

For the strategy options discussed in chapter 2 (payer assessment/ position, physician network assessment/position, organizational and financial capability and performance, merger/alliance position, getting and keeping customers), the same framework for implementation issues can be used.

Payer Involvement

Depending on an organization's goals, the implementation of the payer position might include the following steps:

1. Establish a payer platform for contract negotiations.
2. Develop a contracting vehicle for the range of clinical care services with the affiliated physicians.
3. Consider and prepare for the change in payment systems and the associated medical management issues.
4. Continue to monitor the payer environment.

While refining the specific functions of the contracting vehicle and the change to capitation, the organization should continue to learn about other models for these activities by providing educational programs for the physicians and management. In that way, the strengths and weaknesses of each model become more clear to a group that is learning together, while decision making with a common basis for learning can be achieved in a cooperative atmosphere.

Management should also monitor changes in the marketplace that affect the relevance of the goals. Consolidation in the health care industry affects providers and payers. Changes among payers (mergers with other payers and providers, for example), in addition to their individual performances, may affect the contracting position and terms.

Step 1. Establish a Payer Platform The implementation and management of payer contracts require the following activities:

- developing a platform for contracting for the providers participating in the contracting vehicle
- ensuring that contracts have long-term periods, with long-term termination options and staggered renewal dates
- setting up systems to monitor the status of current contracts, financial items, utilization, medical management, and gains and losses in covered lives

- preparing to change payment modes from discounts to case rates, from per diem rates to global rates
- considering other support structures (information systems reports, capabilities, deal-making capability, and organizational changes to represent the most providers with the most authority)
- continuing to monitor regional markets
- responding to key variables that area regional employers want or developing an action plan to be in position to deliver desired outcomes

The first step in implementation is to establish the payer platform used to negotiate with payers on acceptable terms. The three areas of preparation for a payer platform are establishing minimum, preferred, and average ranges of acceptable contracting standards. Contracting with a platform also ensures parity among payers. The platform should be designed around meeting the goals articulated in the strategic plan. Overall, in addition to the strategy opportunities, the tactical areas for contracting include

- maximizing reimbursement
- increasing and maintaining current volume
- maximizing opportunity for payer determination over clinical decisions and medical management issues

The first step is to maximize reimbursement, while determining what will be required financially for the organization to break even, make regulator-required contributions if or as required, cover the cost of capital, and ensure needed capital replenishment. The organization will strive to have payer-acceptable rates, while covering the required costs to operate the organization. To the extent that the provider-required rates are higher than the market rates, costs of service delivery would have to decrease and efficiencies increase to improve the contracting position.

The range of payer terms can be assessed under different types of payment:

- discounted fee for service
- case reimbursement
- global payments
- shared risk

In the next step, the analysis needs to look at volume reimbursed under several different scenarios to ensure comparability on the payment systems. While the opportunity to increase volume may tempt the organization to offer decreased rates, many of the organizations that have pursued this strategy for the incremental volume found that their reimbursement was less than their cost. In addition to the cost challenge, such a contracting position will, in time, lead other payers to demand rate parity. Another challenge is that the volume apparently brought by a new payer may be converted volume from another payer, rather than new covered lives to the system; therefore, exceptional rates given to new payers for seemingly new volume may be unwarranted discounts. The third challenge is that the favorable rates for new volume, if they are better than existing rates for long-standing relationships, are only going to become modified under another service delivery contract and thus the organization faces a future decrease.

Finally, the opportunity to make determinations on the basis of clinical decisions depends on the clinical resources available. The range of services covered by a single contract (when those services are part of the health care provider) is the primary issue. A secondary issue involves the contract incentive to offer services that are contracted for by the provider. In a marketplace with many nursing homes, contracting for subacute services may be more viable than converting acute care services to subacute services. Having those services available is not always an advantage. Per diem payment terms that are dictated by payers means that an acute admission that is transferred to a subacute unit may have both acute and subacute days denied, based on retrospective review of the patient's health status. Such medical management is in the hands of the payer and not the provider. Global payment terms and care payment terms each put the responsibility for medical management in the hands of the providers.

Cost and value standards from the health care organization should be explored in terms of market standards, best practice standards, and the provider's standards to determine a cost- and value-effective position. The provider with better clinical protocols and briefer lengths of stay has a greater advantage entering into a negotiation than the provider with comparatively less cost-effective care delivery rates.

The payer platform is for the entire set of providers represented, which includes physicians. The payment mechanisms to each provider participant should not sacrifice the financial health of one for the other. The following are necessary action steps:

1. Develop an analytic structure for tolerance for a payer platform, financial structure for payment versus cost and revenue.
2. Determine the parameters of what the physicians can do, and what contracts are of value to employers, to physicians, and to the hospital/delivery system.
3. Assess organizational position, present and future.
4. Review rates (comparatively low or efficient).
5. Compare care delivery.
6. Assess ability to deliver on budget.

7. Calculate cost-efficiency.
8. Determine clinical management ability.
9. Ascertain financial requirements of institution (asking, for example, how low or under what terms an organization can go? Are there gradations of value in payers, based on volume or payment history?).

Ensure that contracts have long-term periods, with long-term termination options. A contract with a short termination notice period for no cause has only secured that financial payment stream as long as the termination clause. In addition, there is merit in staggering contract renewals over time. Staggering transition dates of contracts puts the organization less at risk for change in reimbursement and requires less negotiating activity at the same time.

The payer platform's set of terms may need testing among experts or buyers to ensure that the terms are perceived to have value and will be acceptable.

Step 2. Develop a Contracting Vehicle with or among Physicians

The consolidation of health care organizations has traditionally been attributed to payers. However, professional imaginations have also been fueled during recent debates over health care reform. While this debate has surely highlighted the many options open on the payer side, the options for establishing a vehicle for contracting include management services organizations (MSOs, with managed care contracting as a vehicle), group practice without walls, and physician-hospital organizations (PHOs). Any of these organizational structures that have committed participation by the providers would be feasible for contracting.

Any commitment to a contracting vehicle must be made with the assumption that there is a consensus among the physicians. Prepare for the conversations with the physicians by reviewing the reasons for the contracting entity. Materials may include

- a review of all the managed care products that each of the physicians participates in (likely available through the physician telephone service or a public relations directory)
- a review of all the managed care products in which the acute care provider organization participates
- a summary of how contracting practices by the area managed care organizations prefer to contract (many prefer a simplified contracting vehicle)
- a review of other physician groups, physicians, and hospitals contracting entities in the region
- examples of how contracting together has benefited other physicians or hospitals and the benefits derived from the action

Alignment of the physicians on capitation or risk arrangements requires that the organization:

- establish information systems to give physicians feedback
- further develop and educate physician leadership via
  —the coaching or mentoring of physicians
  —interacting with other participating providers
  —reviewing data and helping set productivity standards and panel size
  —reviewing utilization and help get nonperformers to perform

The organization should review the physicians by specialty in the medical community to determine whether there is a full complement of needed physicians in the services that are offered, and determine what services are missing because of a lack of clinical capabilities. Additionally, management should discuss with the existing medical staff cooperative means to add missing capabilities.

Step 3. Prepare for Changing Modes of Payment: Changing Incentives Consideration of different modes of payments has different implications for medical management. The most dramatic change from the transitions in payment terms is the one to global payments or capitation.

The anticipated move to capitation requires analyzing the existing financial structure of those health care providers participating in the assessment, to determine what the actual health care costs are and what the required reimbursement would be under capitation. This requires actuarial support to develop premium-specific actuarial sound pools using age/sex cells and volume thresholds.

It may be helpful to find a payer with whom there can be a strong partnership in moving toward capitation. Some contracts have stages of volume, or number of "covered lives," in which increasing levels of volume thresholds trip off different payment terms. Three considerations in preparing for capitation are

- having sufficient volume (covered lives) for a risk contract
- having information systems to manage financial and clinical reports on the covered lives in the system
- using actuarial assessment to ensure that both the contract global cap will pay for what is contracted and that the medical community that is part of the contracting has acceptable rates and utilization management background

The challenge is to work with the various providers to engage providers in working together for payment and clinical care issues. The issues to be addressed include

- looking at best practices nationally and regionally
- looking at best practice standards nationally and regionally
- comparing national and regional practices and standards to internal best practices and standards
- determining whether internal best practices are near national, regional, or desired standards
- developing common and goals for accomplishment
- sharing data reports
- setting targets and reviewing progress
- exploring reasons for fewer performers among low performers and developing a target action plan

Leaders should assemble both the decision-making group and the work group and ensure that physicians are involved in the exchange of information that supports recommendations and ultimate decision making. Information on capability (for example, how many covered lives they have, how many visits, utilization information, and so on) must be available to describe the impact on primary care providers, specialists, and hospital services.

The organization should structure the monitoring system(s) to track the status of current contracts, finances, covered lives, utilization, medical management, and gains and losses in covered lives.

The change in payment terms, employer groups, or payment schedules will sharply affect physician practices. While contracts generally have advance notice provisions, the change from short-term admissions to observation status (24-hour care) affects provider revenue budgets.

One payer medical director noted: "Even the onset of observation status replacing admissions in the hospital doesn't slow the rising cost of a hospital stay. Costly multiple invasive procedures, such as cardiac catheterization, can be accomplished on observation status patients that runs up the charges to be as much or more than a full admission."

Of the same payer system another physician noted the change in managing the patient while getting the clinical evaluation done: "The reason to do more testing on shorter-stay patients is to get the full picture by doing concurrent testing rather than sequential testing."

The changes in payment suggest a change in clinical management incentives. The typical practice patterns for health care providers may need to undergo investigation and change. The following is a review of how some organizations are working with affiliated physicians to make changes in preparing for new reimbursement systems:

- Group Health Associates (GHA) in Cincinnati uses continuous quality improvement concepts to change physician behaviors. GHA identifies processes needing improvement and brings together everyone involved in the process. For lower-back pain protocols, primary care physicians, physical therapists, orthopedic specialists, and neurosurgeon met together.

- Morristown (New Jersey) Memorial Hospital relies on data to help boost physician performance. The hospital gets physicians specific clinical performance data from an outside company that takes raw hospital data and generates acuity adjusted reports by diagnosis-related group (DRG) and individual physician. A database integrates medical records and financial data with data from the outside firm. Thus, physicians can see all patient cases within a DRG by medical record numbers, total charges, average charge by cost center, gender, zip code, and the day of the week each admission, procedure, and discharge takes place.

- Salem (Oregon) Hospital uses data to help change physicians' behavior. Variance data are presented on a wall display showing high volume DRGs with significant variations. The chart is in an area provided for physician dictation.

- Phoenix Baptist Hospital and Medical Center uses standing orders to deal with the issues of variation.[6]

The above overview of hospitals preparing their physicians to be aware of their medical management patterns and to consider changes provides a range of approaches to what is becoming a common challenge.

Step 4. Continue to Monitor Payer Trends   The continual monitoring of local and regional payers is essential for keeping pace with actual and potential partners. Moreover, attention should be directed toward changes in Medicare and Medicaid. Such payer changes bring about changes to clinical care management and provider incentives for different types of medical care.

Employers who seek to cut out the middleman are candidates for direct contracting for provider sponsored networks. Self-insured employees are also candidates for provider selection. An example of such an organization follows:

One purchaser that hopes to find success in direct contracting is the Buyers' Health Care Action Group (BHCAG), a Midwestern purchasing coalition that includes such corporate giants as 3M, General Mills Inc., and Honeywell Inc. The Minneapolis-based coalition, which with 250,000 employees will be the largest yet to embrace direct contracting, has begun accepting bids from provider networks such as physician hospital organizations (PHOs) for 50 long-term partial capitation contracts on a uniform set of benefits and will implement the system, which they call the Choice Plus plan, in 1997.[7]

The goals set in establishing an enhanced contracting position with more providers may be achieved through the creation of several vehicles.

Regulations may change to allow or inhibit opportunities for revenue maximization. At the time of this writing, subacute services in hospitals provide a financially lucrative answer for many hospitals' unused acute inpatient beds. However, challenges to Medicare may halt the current cost-based reimbursement for the initial start-up phase, making it a short-lived opportunity. The change in regulations may also allow or halt reporting by organizations, which may change the playing field. Some states regulate HMOs to a greater degree than preferred provider organizations. It is important to keep abreast of regulatory changes and interpretations formally and informally. In addition, there may be opportunities to discuss matters and review public information impacting a particular service area.

Physician Network Development

The drive for offering a full continuum of care has introduced a variety of models for integration that range from varying levels of autonomy to fully merged systems. Although each marketplace differs, additional primary care providers may secure payer contracts, attract more covered lives into a system, and establish a balance to offset a medical community likely dominated by specialists.

Attracting physicians toward integration into a larger system can be accomplished by offering a full spectrum of potential services provided to physicians. These range from the very independent models (entry models) to fully integrated models (ultimate stage models). Figure 5-1 shows some of these models.

Forming a physician network, whatever the model, is being undertaken by most players in the industry. Hospitals form physician networks so that future business can be assured. For-profit physician practice management firms form physician networks to demonstrate efficiencies, leading to climbing price-earning ratios. Payers develop physician networks to ensure access to primary care and other physicians, amassing group strength both to gain payer contracts and to develop practice efficiencies.

Hospitals Hospitals have been acquiring primary care physician practices or investing in them directly in order to secure market share. Hospitals have a long history of developing initiatives to bond with the medical staff in order to increase service use and enhance revenue. By employing primary care physicians, hospitals attract covered lives through managed care channels and respond to some managed care products' requirements for primary care. Although acquiring and managing physician practices is of strategic importance, getting into a new business without adequate expertise and large acquisition prices can result in operating losses. It has been estimated that hospitals lose money on acquired practices about 75 percent of the time.[8] Nevertheless, physician network development has continued to be a growth area for hospitals and IDSs. In a study of employment increases in hospitals from 1981 to 1993, most of the job growth has been in physician offices, where employment grew by 74 percent.[9]

FIGURE 5-1. Spectrum of Services

Entry Models

- *Management services organizations (MSOs).* For a regular fee, MSOs offer billing services, the lease of office space, information systems, group purchasing, group insurance, and recruitment. MSOs are described in more detail at the end of this section.

- *Open physician-hospital organizations (PHOs).* Open PHOs are contracting vehicles for any participating physician with no exclusions. They include shared ownership, shared governance, joint-managed care contracting with the hospital, physicians, and fee-for-service (non-PHO contracts). These include a liberal admission policy and, therefore, the potential for a wrong physician mix. Without controls to make this group cost-effective, payers will not be interested, which will incite the best physicians to leave.

- *Group practices without walls.* These practices share the cost of billing, personnel, purchasing, insurance, and marketing, with a single brand identity and managed care contracting.

Transition Models

- *Closed PHOs.* Closed PHOs offer exclusive contracting for their physicians and selective physician participation. They exclude underperformers and provide stringent reviews of cost and quality performance with performance management and mentoring, and corrected cost and quality performance. This model survives on a long-term basis, as it is more cost-effective; there is a correct mix of specialist and primary care physicians who are appropriately located, all of whom attract payers and more attractive rates, which, in turn, attracts more physicians.

- *Comprehensive MSOs (include payer contracting).* In this scenario, the patients, practice revenues, and contracts are still the physician's. However, the management and contract services are provided at market rates to the participating physicians.

Ultimate Stage Models

- *Foundation model.* Under this model, payment is made to the foundation, which controls the hard practice assets and the patients, practice revenues, and contracts. There may be several group practices overseen by the foundation, which sets individual physician compensation and incentives, and controls practice patterns and physician recruitment.

- *Staff model.* Payment is made to the staff model health system, which distributes the funds to the physicians, sets individual physician compensation and incentives, and controls practice patterns and physician recruitment.

Source: *Health Systems Review* (July/Aug. 1996): 24.

One example of a hospital's early strategic approach to developing a network is noted in figure 5-2, which highlights the importance of quickly entering a market by affiliating with "gold standard" physician practices, instead of taking the time and developing the competence to start a practice.

Physician Practice Management Firms While some physicians have aligned formally with hospitals in establishing their own economic situations, some physicians have preferred to be independent and have joined into loose affiliations known as physician practice management firms (PPMs). The growth of PPMs, especially where physician leadership or physician governance is successful, may provide access to capital and management capabilities otherwise unavailable to independent or small groups of physicians. The firms take over the administrative functions and handle the managed care contract negotiations. Examples of successful PPMs include PhyCor, MedPartners, and Physicians' Quality Care.

Payers Payers with interests in streamlining medical care delivery and aligning incentives among payers, providers, and investors actively moved to acquire and manage physician practices in the early 1990s. The concern over health care reform, which seemed pending in the earlier part of the decade and still looms in one form or another, facilitated the interest in a full scope of health care delivery. Several large insurance companies pursued physician practice acquisition and management for the following purposes:

- to create a seamless delivery of care
- to ensure long-term relationships with providers
- to share risk and reward
- to ensure having a loyal physician base emphasizing primary care
- to have control over physician spending
- to control utilization

FIGURE 5-2. Network Development Approach: University of Chicago Medical Center

1. Partner with the best physicians in target geographies, with the goal of creating managed care group practice enrollment sites.
2. Create a financial contracting and management subsidiary vehicle that can accept and manage prepayment for physician and hospital services.
3. Develop marketable, health plan-oriented practice sites, in conjunction with physician partners.
4. Build the hospital system around the needs of the enrolled population.
5. Build the subacute, home care, and SNF network to complement the clinic and hospital sites.

Source: *GFP Notes 6*, no. 4 (Fall 1993): 19–23, AAMC.

However, with no apparent national reform on the horizon, consumers have few reasons to change physician, when most health plans offer a choice for the same cost savings. As a result, some payers, such as those in the examples below, have changed their physician management strategy:

- FHP International (Fountain Valley, California), which started as a staff-model HMO in 1961, has placed its 500 physicians in a separate company
- Physician Corporation of America (Miami, Florida) agreed to sell 40 medical centers in Florida to FPA Medical Management, which employs 118 primary care physicians and 7 specialists.

Implementing a Physician Network Because of the multiple challenges and new variables that may arise during the implementation process, it is easy to lose the focus on the development of the network when it takes place in a new location. Organizations that have standardized approaches appear to have more success, although their approaches into markets may differ slightly.

The onset of implementation of the physician network position points to activity in the following areas, depending on the statement of the goals:

- *Preparing for a primary care provider network:* See description in following subsection
- *Offering management services to other physicians:* The opportunity to offer management services to other physicians may create savings in the overall operations. For example, the cost of information systems and billing systems is less when shared among more physicians, despite direct costs for each practice.
- *Supporting the medical staff in uniting to form a payer vehicle:* The formation of an independent practice association (IPA) that contracts with payers provides the network with more leverage than physicians would have if they contracted with payers individually.
- *Establishing a forum to have physician leadership and participation in all programs:* The creation of a structure that allows physicians to participate with physician leadership is a hallmark of successful consolidation. Many PPMs cite physician leadership and governance participation as evidence that the new structures are physician controlled.
- *Continuing to monitor and update the physician environment:* In keeping with clinical changes, the creation of systems to increase the efficiency of clinical practice requires continued monitoring and updates. The updates should focus on the needs of physicians and the roles that they play in both overseeing and providing direct care.

Preparing for a Primary Care Provider Network In preparation for physician network development, be sure to clarify the purpose for developing the network. The reasons may include one or more of the following:

- to stabilize an existing primary care physician group to maintain the current source of admissions/covered lives
- to increase the source of admissions/covered lives
- to move further into integration
- to prepare for/respond to payer and employer needs

The process of implementation must keep the purpose in the forefront of all development activities. This process includes

- developing criteria for the physician to affiliate with the network
- setting physician performance and compensation expectations
- identifying the appropriate amount of resources for both capital and acquisition activities
- developing the operational approach for physician practice management
- sealing the deal

Developing criteria for the physician to affiliate with the network: Market opportunities derived from assessing the service area and goals offer a range of choices in criteria for establishing a physician network. One of the key decisions is whether to merge with an existing practice or start a new practice. Similarly, a geographic location must be selected, based on market research of area consumers and existing supply.

Existing practices bring a panel of patients, which means a quicker revenue generation than that of a practice that must attract a panel of patients. In addition, established practitioners may be better mentors to physicians who have come out of training or physicians who are still building their own practices. One urban-based provider, for example, started developing a network, and after the first year had established several centers with newly trained physicians or relocated physicians (from outside the service area). When the provider faced competition from other health care organizations, it shifted its focus to acquiring existing area practices in order to gain panels of patients already affiliated with those physicians. This situation allowed the organization to expand the network without the lead time needed for building the practices.

As the above example illustrates, networks seeking to build market share in a competitive environment benefit from using established practitioners and their patients, which attracts more covered lives. In cases in which the direction of the network development is unclear, the organization uses new physicians, taking the start-up time both to build a panel and to become financially independent.

Once the decision is made to establish a physician network, the network developer faces additional strategic decisions:

- What mechanisms will be used to attract existing physicians?
- What will the physician background selection criteria be?

Because the development of a physician network will likely focus first or eventually on existing practitioners, the network must identify physicians according to the following categories:

- specialty area(s)
- geographic location(s)
- panel size
- practice productivity
- practice capacity

The quality of the network, in the eyes of the consumer, is determined by a patient's relationship with his or her physicians, so good selection of physicians is critical. Relying primarily on technical competence and service quality as its criteria, an organization may use any of the following in selecting a physician:

- education
- training
- board status (board certified or eligible within a set period of time)
- experience
- panel size (that is, the number of patients that identify a physician as their primary care provider)
- commitment (as reflected in job history)
- references

The selection criteria may also include training outside the practice discipline, productivity, clinic capabilities, and relationship skills.

Establishing a minimum and preferred set of criteria for physician selection helps to focus the development of the network. The service standards that will define the access and service capability of the practice may exist in some practices and may be standardized as the network develops.

Setting performance and compensation expectations: The organization should set performance expectations and clarify them in advance. In addition, it should establish the means by which agreed-upon goals may be altered as well as the physician's opportunities for impact. Performance expectations may fall into the categories listed below:

- revenue targets (gross and net)
- visit volume (including the standards for short visits and longer visits, such as physicals)
- panel size
- service standards

Of course, the historic performance of a practice should be reviewed prior to the acquisition or practice merger with the network. However, it should be noted that physician practice earnings tend to show a decrease over the prior year after acquisition.

The impact of the managed care payment schedules, with the change from private practice income to network reimbursement, may necessitate a change in a physician's policies and practices. And a physician may be unclear about the organization's expectations regarding productivity based on revenue targets, visits volume, and panel targets. These expectations should be discussed as specifically as possible prior to the acquisition/merger with a network.

Physician compensation is subject to legal scrutiny. Guidelines warn about overpayment for physician practices as well as the types of incentives allowable. While it is important to match prior earnings while guaranteeing most or all of prior income, it is also important to be aware of the most recent reports.

Identifying appropriate amount of resources: After a purpose is delineated and clinicians designated, the organization must ensure adequate resources to develop the network. The amount of capital required to invest in existing physician practices, as well as that needed to start physician practices, varies throughout the country and an organization must consider both the legal and marketplace atmosphere carefully.

Consider the steps needed for starting up as opposed to maintaining an existing management:

1. Determine acquisition resources and resource allocation between acquisition and management.
2. Decide payment terms for assets.
3. Delineate payment value goodwill (may use discounted net present value analysis) or stipend/bonus for starting.
4. Ascertain accounts receivable disposition.
5. Determine the financial requirements to initiate or grow a primary care physician network through start-ups and acquisition.

In addition to the payer contract negotiations, decisions regarding real estate and the most efficient means of practice also affect the physician practice. Whether to obtain a short-term or long-term lease, or to purchase the real estate, will need consideration with regard to potential shifts in land value and the success of the practice. A short-term lease, for example, might mean a potentially large price increase at the term's conclusion, while it also allows the option of another provider taking over the lease. The legal guidelines do require demonstrated market pricing and regular updates as to market prices for physician compensation and market factors.

Developing the operational approach for physician practice management: Physician consolidation takes many forms. The operational approach to leadership, decision-making processes, resource allocation, and day-to-day management should be defined before making any final decision. It should also be compared to the existing operational parameters so that the advantages and disadvantages are clear.

Sealing the deal: Before negotiating with physicians, a new organization must be prepared, demonstrating knowledge of the general marketplace as well as of the physicians' competition, consumers/patients, and payers and sources of revenues. In short, prospective employers must tell a physician as much about their own situations as they know and more. A compelling argument for the future success of the network will be based on solid market research and strategic planning.

When possible, make recommendations for the physician's financial success (revenues and expenses) and describe the proposed process for productivity (expected workload, support resources, and expansion options). Emphasize the long-term relationships and model contracts, including incentives.

Transition from Entrepreneur to Network Member The shift from small private practice to part of a group can have a great impact on many areas of a practice. First, the decision-making process concerning new expenses, personnel, and payment policies that affect everyday life in a practice becomes part of a system that may to a new member seem inflexible. Second, the systems through which administrative policies are developed or altered are new, affecting management, information systems, finances, staff personnel issues, operations, and marketing activities; decisions about service standards and productivity for all people who work at a practice are made outside the practice at a larger group level. The more flexible the operational changes are, the easier the transition.

The Friendly Hills Healthcare Network (now part of MedPartners), a leading integrated health care system in Southern California, uses a variety of techniques for helping physicians acclimate to practicing in a managed care organization, including

- physician education, in which day-to-day methods and policies necessary to survive in today's environment (ordering fewer tests, making few referrals to specialists, and so on) are related

- mentors, made available to help colleagues work in a managed care environment
- appropriate compensation and rewards for productivity, participation in leadership activities, cost-effective patient care, and member satisfaction
- feedback via clear performance measures to help physicians understand expectations regarding their performance
- support systems of service professionals, such as pharmacists and case managers
- management participation and appointing qualified physicians to key management positions[10]

Establishing a primary care provider network affects the rest of the medical staff. In cases in which private practice physicians perceive favoritism toward the employed physicians, the provider, in effect, competes with other physicians. The loyalty of those physicians may start to weaken, in light of the employed physicians who are able to benefit from the largess of the hiring organization.

In such cases, the management service organization (MSO) may become a viable vehicle in providing management support while the physicians retain autonomy in private practice. In addition, the PHO, as a contracting vehicle, may provide marketing support in attracting and keeping customers through private contracting with payers.

Offering Management Services to Other Physicians MSOs are established to provide management and administrative services to physicians, hospitals, and other health care providers. MSOs can be an important part of a decentralized health care delivery system, linking each practice's management and the common support systems. Joining an MSO allows clinical independence for a physician, because the MSO handles the administrative side of the practice. MSOs offer solutions for physicians who prefer to retain their autonomy and independence, while still having professional management services.

Although generally viewed as beneficial from the physician's perspective, MSOs are considered a middle-of-the-road integration strategy and not a fully integrated consolidation of health care providers as are PHOs or merged clinics and hospitals.

Nevertheless, services, such as accounting, billing, coding, collections, computer support, legal advice, marketing, payroll processing, and management expertise are generally available for a monthly fee through MSOs, and one example of the successful creation of an MSO for such purposes follows:

Metropolitan MSO in Grand Rapids started in 1993 by eight osteopaths, funded through Metropolitan Hospital. In 1995, there were 26 physicians representing 18 practices, 13 of them primary care. The executive board includes four physicians and four hospital executives. On physician revenue matters, the doctors' votes are counted as 51 percent. The MSO was set up to reduce overhead and establish an organization quickly because of the geographic spread through an urban area. Remaining independent was important and the group was not ready to form a group practice without walls. All the practices are on the same computer system partly because of the objective to become competitive as a physician organization and, therefore, needing claims information for health plans or employers.[11]

Still, problems may arise from employing MSOs without the coding and collections expertise of a physician practice. In addition, if the hospital-sponsored MSO is more interested in maintaining its own solvency than developing true partnerships with the physicians, then the physicians' conflicting agendas come to the forefront.

The generic benefits of joining an MSO, seen more as a short-term solution to developing a fully integrated delivery system, include

- increasing income (both through increasing revenue and reducing costs)
- increasing managed care contracting influence
- improving a practice lifestyle by decreasing management responsibility
- dealing effectively with increasing regulations
- increasing control over practice
- providing an option for participation in corporate policies
- allowing access to capital
- retaining autonomy
- participating in strategic and operational management

The requirements for successful MSOs include the presence of actual management expertise in financial and systems management, as well as active physician participation in governance and operational decision making.

Organizational and Financial Capabilities

Attention to organizational and financial issues is essential to the network implementation process. The clinical service delivery, regardless of the level of care provided, faces change driven by payers, innovations in care delivery, and the need to differentiate one service from other area services.

These changes must be supported by the infrastructure of the organization. The assimilation of strategies affects finance, facilities, human resources, and marketing, and some of the modifications needed to support new strategic initiatives include

- operational enhancements
- creative or strategic use of fiscal services
- facilities used for strategic advantage
- access to information systems
- human resources changes to develop training, employee selection processes, and performance management systems

Operational Enhancements A variety of organizational enhancements may be made in establishing a provider network. One example is to enhance such key service specialties as cardiology, oncology, women's health, pediatrics, and emergency services.

The identification of clinical services by specialty continues as the focus for physician training as well as hospital admission. Although services at a network may need strengthening in certain areas, they also may require modification to accommodate a broader level of integration, including employed physicians and their office practices, state of the art diagnostic and prevention capability, and treatment and rehabilitation capability.

Moreover, clinical services undergoing review or modification may need strengthening or modifying in the context of a different payment system. Under capitation or fee for service, the mode of health care delivery would suggest that both prevention and follow-up support services may be needed to offset the traditional inpatient and outpatient services. In fact, establishing a full spectrum of care may necessitate the following steps:

1. Organize a small group of relevant clinicians and staff to work on the service enhancement or modification. It is important to involve the formal and informal leaders invested in the clinical service, with the understanding, that when complete, the formal leadership will oversee the implementation and monitor the new service. The service-line development process needs a champion who will be innovative within the organization. The service line champion is the person who sees both the potential for integrating more creative applications of the service and the specific steps needed to get the work done.
2. Evaluate the current service by charting the services offered in the actual organization, and then by the affiliated organization(s).
3. Review what services are available in nonaffiliated organizations that would fill any gaps. If there are multiple service providers, then there is an opportunity to develop a service or establish an affiliation, based on clinical, service, and financial criteria.

4. Review the coordination and referral services to determine whether there is a way to enhance coordination and reduce duplication of services.

5. Assure that the quality, cost, and configurations for customer interests are up to the standards of the payers, the users, and the referrers, as well as differentiation standards.

6. Establish monitoring standards and ongoing oversight to make sure the service is progressing as planned. Before the service-line team is disbanded, oversight responsibilities should be assigned to a member of the existing staff as a means of getting him or her involved and responsible for the service.

In addition, gathering information about state-of-the-art treatment for each service line is important in creatively and efficiently refining a service line.

Creative or Strategic Use of Fiscal Services   One of the first steps in integrating the plan into the ongoing life of the organization is through the operating budget process, which is usually started during the strategy development process. It is likely that financial viability criteria have already been applied to most projects at this point, and will continue to be considered in the service-specific initiatives. The existing financial scenarios need to be revisited to account for the costs and benefits of the initiatives and assessed for their impact on the overall financial picture. Any core service development or refinement will have a cost and revenue implication, which should also be assessed and included in the overall budget.

Since the general pursuit of health care organizations is to get and keep customers, accessing customers through payer contracts means that the fiscal service area must work to integrate payers and prepare for capitation. If the operation of managed care development is a separate function, the focus on charges and collection according to contract terms remains an issue that the financial organization will need to manage closely.

In general, the fiscal services division's challenges in responding to the strategic plan are

- revising budget and reimbursement approaches based on staged strategic initiative completion
- preparing for payer contracting with fiscal tools for cost efficiency and preparing for capitation, if relevant
- managing the approach to the overall systemwide businesses, including the hospital, physician practices, managed care products, and related services
- considering potentially cost-effective activities relevant to other financial resources or from other services based on merger or alliance
- understanding the costs and financial benefits of the initiatives growing out of the plan's implementation

To the extent that the financial management of each of the entities or multiple sites are duplicated, there may be an opportunity to decrease costs, which will lead to combining some operations. According to Stephen Shortell and David Anderson, who completed a four-year study of integration paths of 11 regional health systems, "By linking economically with doctors and coordinating finance . . . and other support areas, health system executives can begin to grasp the bigger payoff of clinical integration."[12]

In a recently released report of the *1996–1997 Almanac of Hospital Financial and Operating Indicators,* authored by William O. Cleverley and published by the Center of Healthcare Industry Performance Studies, the hospital industry's financial condition has never been better, as overall profitability has improved and costs are under control.[13] However, a widening gap between high and low performers was projected. Small urban hospitals, in the worst shape of any sector, expected more mergers or affiliations with major facilities in their markets as well as outright closures and bankruptcies among those hospitals with significant debt.[14]

Regarding the generation of hospital funds, one article noted:

> Successful hospitals will be the ones . . . aggressively building up assets for the long term. . . .The hospital will have several dedicated, single purpose funds, each designed for a specific need [such as a] charitable fund for indigent patient care, another fund for capital expenses, a fund for purchase of physicians' practices, a research and education fund, a fund for repair and replacement of operating equipment, a debt reserve fund, building fund, gift giving fund and so on. The hospital may also have an endowment or foundation to build further ties to the community during the annual capital development campaign.[15]

Facilities Used for Strategic Advantage Facilities have taken on a different role in the evolving health care environment. Previously, the most cherished and key asset of health care delivery organizations—the bricks and mortar—can now as easily be regarded as a liability, and an especially inflexible one. Although some organizations are investing heavily in their physical facilities, others are divesting to more nimbly deploy resources. Overall the role of facilities is changing dramatically as a more social model of health care is established, which is resulting in more outpatient modalities and home care. Thus, the previously paid-for hospital inpatient facility has decreased in funding priority, making way for the acquisition of the primary care network.

The facilities division's primary purposes in driving the strategic plan are to

- enable facility upgrade and accommodation of staged strategic initiative completion
- prepare for payer pressure on more outpatient or physician practice capacity, enhancing maximum throughput and cost efficiency

- ensure facility accommodation of inpatient, outpatient, and supplemental services needs and programs
- enable potential consolidation of activities as needed with other facilities from other organizations, as mergers or alliances denote changing of services

Access to Information Systems   Access to decision-making information has brought to the forefront the importance of information systems, replacing the previously pivotal focus on facilities in cost-based reimbursement. In the increasingly competitive arenas of managed care, capitation, and physician practice alliances, information—whether on the organization itself or its potential competitors and collaborators—will be a distinguishing element. Having the right systems and technology in place can give the health care organization a competitive edge. One example of a successful information system is Henry Ford Health System in Detroit:

> Henry Ford Health System's four hospitals and two medical groups expect to have completed a new information systems that provides lab and radiology results, billing information and clinical financial details to a central database. . . . Not only will the system create greater convenience for patients—one medical record and one bill . . . but it will keep its 'clinical policies' on line and in use.[16]

A 1996 Ernst and Young survey on integrated delivery and financing systems noted the following categories of information system capabilities:

- utilization information
- critical pathways
- length of stay
- case management
- auto criteria
- remote dial
- produce Health Plan Employer Data and Information Set (HEDIS) data
- free text[17]

Information systems have applications in the following areas:

- *Aspects of care delivery other than acute care.* Information systems play a critical role in the transition from acute care hospital service delivery to including other aspects of care delivery. At a minimum, changes in systems will need to be made, even if only to avoid duplication of information gathering on customers from the physician office for the ancillary services, for the scheduling of surgery, for the emergency department use, for discharge planning proposes, and for the service registration for after acute care discharge. To the extent that physician group practices align with larger systems and share capitated payments, the scope of care provided elsewhere is critical for their own management and for their productivity. Information systems can allow greater access for the primary care provider, thus preventing time delays in getting information about patients, delaying patient care decisions. As clinical protocols cover the scope of pre-hospital care, acute care services, and postacute care discharge (whether a subacute service or home care protocols), the information about the customer needs to move with the customer.

- *Ensuring operational quality.* In other organizations the investment in and use of information systems is the means of ensuring operational quality. Although this has been a long-debated topic, the "art" of medicine, which has been the focus of medical care delivery, has quietly considered the use of computer technology to automate clinical conclusions and leave the final review for the physicians.
- *Plans for expansion.* The Carle Health Care System, located in Urbana, Illinois, has a 300-bed hospital and 280 physicians. Carle has been an integrated health care system for 15 years. Its strategic plan is focused on the expansion of market share, the building and expansion of clinic, and expansion of the system's out-of-hospital business, all within the purview of the Carle Foundation: "The strategic plan also includes substantial new investments in an already advanced information network . . . making it possible to spread expenses over a larger market while enhancing revenue opportunity. The system is moving to electronic medical records."[18]
- *Job design and clinical quality.* Another application of information technology, in addition to management of patients and clinical management, is the use of information technology on job design and clinical quality. According to Dr. Richard Shea, vice president of medical affairs at Morton Plant Mease Health Care in Florida, work groups are able to track their progress using a computerized template that standardizes the presentation of the measurement tools throughout the health system. In addition to the regular quality training for their 6,000 employees, this technology can bring continuous improvement to the team member level—where it is reviewed at least monthly by the team leader or director.[19]

Not surprisingly, systems changes that are this wide in scope will not come easily. Substantial preparation during the planning exercise, focused on aligning technology with business goals, will facilitate required prioritization of any systems initiatives. With so many opportunities for systems enhancements, implementations, and consolidations, the successful health care organization will focus its systems efforts in those areas where they will have the greatest strategic effect.

Human Resources Changes It has been said of companies known as leaders in customer service that "They pay extraordinary attention to their employees. . . . These companies minimize turnover, the bane of good service, with an impressive array of motivational and training programs. In the interest of increasing customer satisfaction, they give their employees lavish awards and genuine opportunities for advancement."[20]

In order to provide good customer service, employees must clearly understand their own part in the success of the organization; this better enables them to satisfy the customer, without whom no one would have a job.

Most organizations facing a major shift in strategy or focus expect employees to invest themselves in the changes. To this end, in an industry facing dramatic change, employees need to be knowledgeable about and participate in the organization's financial situation. Methods can range from profit-sharing incentives to significant committee structure, such as an adoption of the Scanlon Plan at Boston's Beth Israel Hospital to engage the employees in the organization and make real efforts at meaningful change.

Boston's Beth Israel Hospital (now Beth Israel Deaconness Medical Center) saw the real gain in an initiative to implement the Scanlon Plan of participative management. The program, now in its ninth year at Beth Israel, is called Prepare 21 (to prepare for the twenty-first century). In this system, teams of professionals come together to resolve work problems, and all employees are invited to make cost-saving suggestions. In the early stages of measurement, this system saved over $1 million, with less than 30 percent of that as a start-up cost. However, the longer the plan has been in place, the less decipherable the savings have become, since the organization's culture incorporated the whole aspect of participation and cost reduction as a means of doing business. This underscores the opportunity that exists to solve financial and operational problems with a properly motivated and managed workforce.

Successfully shifting the efforts of a workforce in strategically different directions—and potentially into different jobs—requires proper training and resources. Training not only shows commitment to employees, it is a requirement for producing an adept workforce able to respond to strategic opportunities. Providing motivation and reward systems that will encourage a workforce to face strategic change calls for modern performance management systems.

The pressures of downsizing and the trend of reengineering dramatically change job requirements in a work environment. These changes may be aided by using new technology, reducing the learning curve, and offering new programs and more interdisciplinary team work to resolve service issues.

An organization should anticipate change and determine how staff will best be refocused or redeployed, rather than being forced to resort to layoffs. A strategy anticipating changes is more readily accepted by a workforce when management considers potential job changes and starts cross-training and finding other uses for job skills. Anticipating change may prove particularly challenging for an organization that is not properly prepared for the shift from a disease-oriented care model to a total health care model.

COLLABORATIVE MARKETING

Implementation of any strategic plan in an environment as interdependent as health care requires developing new approaches to collaborative marketing. The keys to success in this area will come not only in traditional and nontraditional marketing, but in creating alliances to extend the organization's ability to acquire and keep customers.

Marketing

The planning cycles for marketing activities should move from an annual to a continuous planning cycle with ongoing reviews of data. Some of the activities that should be included in review sessions include

- establishing benchmarks against world class and regional competitors
- keeping current on other key providers
- looking at new events and responding appropriately
- making sure to be flexible and open to new entrants

As implementation of health care delivery strategy progresses, the opportunity to move from option to option rapidly is essential for success. Once the strategic mix has stabilized, then defined added-value mechanisms can be clarified and communicated. In the wake of consolidation and rapid market change, it is important to keep the service-delivery staff aware of resources in the system. As a labor intensive business, with many points of contact with consumers, using employees to affect member services is critical.

Moreover, to keep current on marketing activity, the development of process teams, product teams, and customer teams may also prove useful. Successful collaborative marketing results depend on established marketing activities that involve

- payers
- service array
- community benefit and collaboration
- promotion

Payers Marketing the relationship of and with the payers is important in considering the actual covered lives and moving from mathematical projection to real attainment. The measure of assessment and market work includes

- comparing actual enrollment to expected enrollment by geographic area and by account type (employer or public program)
- measuring actual access to the marketplace through the payer contracts and looking at their market penetration by employer
- measuring the specific payer enrollees by affiliated primary care physician
- measuring a plan's success in service area (for use in later negotiation) by the above measures and independent utilization and market research

Marketing the consolidated medical community includes not only the right mix of physicians geographically and according to training and speciality, but also the presentation of physician practices in terms of service standards. Promoting ease in accessing a practice initially or for follow-up care, as well as the quality of support of its staff, are becoming a standard among networks seeking to differentiate themselves from the traditional, and often more difficult to use, physician office practices. Such concerns are illustrated below:

> Pennsylvania Blue Cross is establishing several medical centers and facilities in the Allegheny area, in which established physicians, with whom they partner, will move their practices. The basis of developing these service models is market research on the preferences of service users with the findings that support staff have to be caring and friendly, the access to the physicians has to be simplified and the medical service centers have more services available, such as full testing services. In addition, nurses will be available on off hours both to answer questions and to schedule follow up visits in physicians schedules.[21]

Moreover, the onset of value-driven, physician-oriented services has shifted public focus beyond mere access to physicians toward the transition from providing medical service delivery to providing health care resources.

Service Array Modifications to a system of available services will make an organization more market-responsive to direct users, to physicians, and to payers. Intertwined with the formation of services that range across several modes of clinical delivery is the need to keep the customer educated and ensure that service modifications are evident. Areas in which modifications may be directed include

- a revised role for emergency services in a managed care environment
- the use of nursing staff, who can schedule follow-up appointments, 24 hours a day
- the presence of a staff person to help with both the payer and primary care physician selection and authorization in primary care practice offices and centers
- more support groups and well health care programs

Community Benefit and Collaboration The demonstrated value of health care organizations toward serving the community, while inherent in many founding missions and present in many services, bears revisiting amidst pressure to be more business-oriented.

The consolidation of health care delivery systems and the payer's demand for a less fragmented system highlights the need for actual collaboration with community service providers in the interest of improved health care delivery. Developing a broader health care referral and coordination system both ensures a seamless delivery of care and starts a virtual or actual partnership that may become contractual under capitation. By not duplicating services, the local collaboration will in the long run reduce costs to the health care system. Acute care and long-term care facilities that coordinate delivery of respite services can provide such services at the least cost. For example, facilities may accept Medicare patients discharged from acute care facilities on Fridays, instead of sending them home without state-supported services over the weekend.

Such commitment to the community complements the traditional network mission statement of responding to local needs. Heightened attention to healthier communities and relationships with schools, social service agencies, and other providers are manifestations of the partnerships that help a hospital respond to its mission.

Examples of ways in which health care organizations can reach out to their communities are described below.

- The Virginia coalition, from the University of Virginia Medical Center, has targeted eight outreach areas, including immunization, teen pregnancy, and improving low-income women's access to breast cancer exams. The goal is to develop long-term community relationships.
- At Veterans Memorial Medical Center in Meriden, Connecticut, hospital officials are developing a policy that would require all

managers and professional staff to be involved in community activities; part of the annual performance review would consider how well an individual has met that goal.

- Kaiser Permanente in Vallejo, California, in an initiative directed toward three low-income neighborhoods, has determined the most efficient use of hospital resources includes a team of nurses, community health outreach specialists, and residents who are trained to help remove the barriers that inhibit access.

- To improve service to Medicaid patients, PMH Health Services Network in Phoenix (a system of Phoenix Memorial Hospital, an HMO and a group practice of physicians) opened six school-based health centers that offer a wide range of services and help erode the distrust that many of the area's Latino population feel toward hospitals.[22]

Overall, the community benefit or healthier community initiative should be selected based on indicated local needs. Once the need is identified, the forum for responding to that need should be explored. Some of the opportunities to effect healthier communities may include

- shared clinical education and outreach
- joint projects on clinical education
- issues for public concern supported by incidence data
- joint feasibility studies
- public education programs

There are many examples of how cooperative services are developed with local service agencies who play different roles in the lives of those needing support and services. These include

- joint planning with schools leading to health education or on-site medical care
- joint planning with town or city health staff, promoting public health issues as the responsibility of all parties
- cooperative feasibility studies involving social service outreach
- shared public education programs with agencies, such as an American Heart Association program on chest pain management or a shared campaign for child safety
- repackaging physician-written articles for community social service agencies for educational purposes

In short, an investment in the community initiates community partnerships and serves as a model for more involvement and support. Collaboration avoids cost increases resulting from an institution recreating locally available services and adds value to the community.

Promotion In the wake of consolidation, having meaningful, results-oriented promotions is important to break through what may be a confusing set of communications from health care delivery organizations amidst great change. As the organization changes scope, name, and focus, the first major component of promotion is to keep key groups informed.

Keeping key constituents informed is important in retaining loyalty and keeping relationships intact. It is imperative, for example, to keep employees, donors, and key advisors abreast of mergers or network affiliations before such occurrences are noted in the local media. Information about a merger or consolidation that might come to the attention of the press can be the subject of simultaneous correspondence, via E-mail or memos, to donors and employees, ensuring that those connected with the organization are notified from inside the company and retain their loyalty.

The second major component is to keep communication lines open with existing and new user groups about the changes in an organization. Changes in leadership, name identification, and systems that provide new avenues of accessing a service require a complete communication plan that is sequenced to respond to current users, new users, current service delivery staff (employees), and new service delivery staff (new or potential employees).

Having formatted an organization's offerings into user-friendly services, the network may employ the media mix of press releases, events, advertisements, and direct mail all at once or individually, using strategic messages in consumer-friendly language. Meaningful, results-oriented promotions might include direct-response promotions, allowing an organization's reach to be measured.

The measures for evaluating success in a promotion are based on direct response or actual volume changes. Further, market research on aided and unaided public awareness and the changes in a customer's willingness to try the service will also provide feedback. Cooperative promotion of facilities within a network, with common endorsements, sends a message of uniformity. Even events to build traffic into areas around new primary care service centers or physician offices make a difference.

Creation of Alliances

Alliance activity has been touted as the best means to consolidate an overcrowded industry (burdened with too many fixed assets and declining utilization) and to achieve strategically necessary efficiencies. It is also the heart of collaborative marketing efforts.

Driven by the goals of decreasing expenses, increasing managed care contracts, increasing market share, and improving the ability to boost community health status, providers pooling their resources and knowledge is an important example of services working together to enhance services to the consumer. Collaboration may be essential for organizations to achieve more attractive positions for the long-term in their marketplaces and to improve service delivery. One example of such an alliance follows:

> Blue Cross and Blue Shield of Maryland plans to invest in and take over the marketing of a provider sponsored managed care company. Blue Cross is banking on its initial stake on the potential for a stepped-up marketing effort to improve the enrollment. The marketing and distribution force is 10 times the size of the managed care company (Preferred Health Network [PHN]) and most likely will promote the plan to small work forces of less than 200 employees that value choice. If the strategy works, PHN will gain the increased patient flow while the Blues plan profits from growth through increased value of its 16 percent share plus an as-yet-undetermined percentage of revenues as a marketing fee.[23]

Affiliations and Consolidations   Affiliations should be pursued with clear-cut reasons and objectives, as they take time and resources, and may have limited outcomes. With the increasing payer-motivated call to decrease costs and streamline health care, merger and alliance activity has been strong in the last several years.

According to *Modern Healthcare*, mergers and acquisitions hit a pace of 2.4 per day among all types of providers in the first half of 1996. Among hospitals alone, one deal every three days has occurred in the past 2.5 years, many involving multiple facilities, according to Irving Levin Associates of New Canaan, Connecticut. One fifth of community hospitals changed hands in 1994 and 1995.[24]

There are mixed reactions to the enormous amount of alliance activity. In a full-asset merger, establishing a new organization requires an unknown amount of resources to achieve the expected results. That invites the criticism that health care consolidation is more focused on amassing power by enlarging a total asset base than on the expected outcomes. Missed market signals, resulting in strategic surprises, become further evidence that short-term gains are not realized in the structuring of an industry. Despite the strategic drive for a physician network, the operating losses from acquired physician practices (or long-term break-even time frames) have prompted HMOs to sell physician practices or hospitals bringing in for-profit management companies to stem the losses. Although consolidation has brought and is bringing together medical care resources in a national vision of integrated health systems, the expected outcomes may not be readily apparent. Consolidation among pharmaceutical companies, for example, raises the following points: "The 10 largest drug companies' average United States revenues almost doubled from 1990–1995, largely due to mergers, but their total market share grew only five percentage points to about 52%. This raises the possibility that the rest of the industry outperformed them, although companies' performance can be evaluated in many ways."[25]

Consolidation in health care delivery requires difficult decision making among organizations that need a consensus to manage overall. Layering in another organization may compromise the strategic vision, without a real focus on the expected and actual outcome. Critics argue that seven percent of surveyed organizations reduced or eliminated patient services in the last two years since merging or being acquired.[26]

Revenue and Market Share Considerations Increasing or stabilizing revenue and market share are driving factors for consolidation. Becoming attractive to payers is a means of both securing market share and increasing revenue. As a driving factor, three systems, described below, are proceeding to explore ways of decreasing cost and increasing revenues and contracts.

> In early fall of 1996, three of North Carolina's largest not-for-profit health care systems [Carolinas Health Care System, North Carolina Baptist Hospital, and Pitt County Memorial Hospital] were discussing an alliance that would involve coordinating services and jointly pursuing service contracts with payers. The goal of the alliance would be to reduce health care costs by undertaking joint projects, avoiding duplicative services, sharing administrative and support services and pursuing managed care opportunities.[27]

Alliances that leave core assets in place while expanding across state borders are also being developed. Following are three examples of cross-border alliances:

- Lahey-Hitchcock Medical System is a merger of the New Hampshire based Mary Hitchcock Hospital and associated medical group as well as the Massachusetts Lahey Clinic and associated hospital.
- Cooley Dickenson Hospital developed an affiliation with the Hitchcock Medical Group before the system moved more fully into Massachusetts with the Lahey merger.
- Presbyterian Hospital, the patient care arm of New York's Columbia Presbyterian Medical Center, intends to expand its managed care contracting network through a corporate partnership with Palisades Medical Center in New Jersey's Hudson County, as the first corporate linkage of New York City and New Jersey. It is only a bridge affiliation; each organization will have control of its own assets, as a result of Palisades Hospital wanting a high degree of local control and involvement in the local community.[28]

Strategic Considerations for Pursuing an Alliance Potential goals in pursuing an alliance include

- enhanced services offerings
- expanded referral sources
- economies of scale
- capacity to structure delivery system and allocate resources
- improved access to capital
- improved debt capacity
- integration of all essential systems elements (underwriting, provision of services, administration)
- allowance for a systems approach to care delivery, utilization review, resource allocation, and pricing
- allowance for flexibility in pricing and service arrangements
- hospital or PHO control of the system
- primacy of provider perspective in the formation of the system

In considering the strategies of national provider firms, their focus is clearer, because it is more universal, although applied differently in each regional marketplace. Overall, Columbia/HCA, for example, seeks "to decrease hospital costs by converting purchasing to national contracts and eliminating some fixed assets, while spreading remaining high fixed costs over other providers and securing a larger patient base. Overall, Columbia/HCA strengthens its market position to share services, to decrease cost, and to bid for provider contracts with managed care organizations."[29]

Complete, successful alliances or mergers are similar in that each partner shares a common vision of the future as well as complementary capabilities. Consider figure 5-3, which reviews the assessment of the organizations, when evaluating a potential partner. Shared goals for the future will help each organization further the alliance, while acknowledged strengths brought to the partnership will bolster the capabilities of the whole.

In figure 5-4, the process of proceeding with an alliance is delineated: reviewing the purpose of an alliance, looking at all potential partners, developing the relationship structure, developing the deal, and establishing either a team management or merging cultures. This process is followed by actual operation through integration or initiation and concludes with the monitoring of results.

Organizations may need to consider several partner options. To find both the partner and structure for an alliance requires focus. The new partner must be willing and able to adopt the organization's purpose, or the affiliation will be without value. Because of the potential pitfalls in the partner-exploration process, an organization should draw up a list of potential suitors and explore several options concurrently. As an example,

FIGURE 5-3. Checklist for Alliance Partner Candidates

Checklist of key factors in shopping for alliance partner

1. Shared assumption about the environment or shared vision of the drivers affecting the future
2. Shared vision for health care delivery
3. Complementary strengths
4. Comparison of the key aspects of the organization that result in shared notions about duplication, similarity, or complementary capabilities when comparing
   - payer position
   - physician network
   - financial position
   - organizational performance and services
   - position on alliances
   - getting and keeping customers

WellPoint's partnership discussions take place continually throughout the country:

> WellPoint has a strategy of buying insurance companies that seek to exit the health care business. WellPoint eases their indemnity clients into more profitable managed-care products (such as the group health insurance subsidiary of Mass Mutual Life Insurance). WellPoint isn't focusing on HMOs but on creating products tailored to specific customer need, offering a wide variety of products from indemnity plans to HMO hybrids. To meet those goals, WellPoint plans to acquire companies and build products from scratch. There are continual discussions with potential partners all over the country, including other BC/BS plans.[30]

The checklist contained in Figure 5-5 shows the types of issues that are considered during the discussions of the actual alliance.

Structure of an Alliance Based on the axiom form follows function, the structure of the alliance should mirror the actual intent of the organization's activities. Therefore, a review of the goals and expected outcomes shapes the relationship structure. Relationship structures are informed by the answers to the following questions:

- What should be accomplished?
- What should not occur?
- When is it time to walk away?

Based on what can and cannot be accomplished within the scope of an alliance, the structure of the alliance and a relationship then takes

FIGURE 5-4. Checklist for Partnership/Alliance Considerations

1. *What is the purpose of the alliance?*

   What do we need from an alliance?

   What would we bring to an alliance?

   The purpose of an alliance should be the same on both sides, although supporting benefits to each participant may differ. If the purpose of the alliance differs for both sides, operationalizing will be a problem because both sides would resolve the issues differently, each according to its purpose.

2. *What is the line of business of the alliance?*

   It should be more than a familiarity of philosophies about the business or the future. There should be clear-cut functional reasons for coming together, where concrete actions would likely be taken or the effort of coming together will have no result.

3. *Who are the candidates for alliances?*

   Assuming that the goal can be accomplished by different resources. There may be more than one suitable partner to achieve an outcome, which may be pursued concurrently or sequentially (in order of priority).

4. *What are the criteria for selecting the final candidate for an alliance?*

   This may include consistent organizational values. Compatibility in values will assist the shaping of a common vision and combining organizational culture. Values compatibility may preclude other organizations that would bring complementary benefits to the organization, such as leadership or board transition. Some mergers cannot continue with direction from both parties on leadership transition, such as operating priorities of the alliance, capital contribution, resource allocation from each side, the criteria allowing the alliance to dissolve and who gets the alliance owned assets, the level of flexibility among the candidates and the level of access to other.

5. *What is the method for establishing alliance?*

   There should be a recognized process of establishing an alliance that is set for the organization in advance so that they will not inadvertently lose opportunities or a position that would be regretted later.

6. *What are the strengths of each participant in an alliance?*

   Each organization's strengths should be listed, from the perspective of financial capability, market draw, differentiating capabilities, organizational culture, and adaptability to work with another organization.

7. *Risks/Costs*

   These are items to consider in establishing an alliance:

   - With the alliance, are we stronger long term to the customer base? (focusing on recruitment and/or retention)
   - Are we a stronger player (compared to the competitors) in the market?
   - Are we potentially losing market advantage that we currently enjoy/have?
   - Are we losing current benefits of operating alone by having this alliance?

FIGURE 5-4. *(Continued)*

8. *Cultural issues to understand and consider in the allied business*

   Cultural orientation of each participant expressed in the following ways:

   - Decision making (how and who has the final authority to make things happen in the organization and at what level)
   - Focus of resources (where are the resources or new resources generally focused
   - Criteria for prior expansion/divestment (what is the criteria for how key strategic services have been expanded or divested?)
   - Centralized versus decentralized level of decision making and what the basis is for who can make what kinds of decisions

9. *Resources needed to pursue alliance*

10. *Intended outcome of the alliance:*

    - Criteria for success
    - Threshold for failure/dissolution
    - The "out" terms and who gets the shared resources/risks when the break-up comes

---

shape. The structure of the relationship might include any of the following options:

- cooperative ventures/joint planning
- shared services
- service trade and partnerships
- affiliations, alliances, and networks
- mergers and acquisitions

Assessing opportunities offered by merger activity: The merger activity in the health care delivery and payer industry has a range of opportunities. Most industry observers agree that unless the local and regional markets are actually part of the development of integration, integration is meaningless. This may call for educating the purchasers about opportunities available for increased value in the formulation of an alliance or an integrated health care delivery system, or it may call for a slower development by the health care provider or payer before the amalgamation of full-scale integration. One recent set of discussions allows for any type of alliance, from a full-asset merger to limited alliances on specific courses of business:

> Kaiser Permanente Unit and Group Health Cooperative of Puget Sound have entered discussion that could lead to a merger. . . . The move illustrates the threat posed to the nonprofit sector of the health-care industry by the growing dominance of investor-owned companies that can more easily finance expansion and operational improvements because of their access to capital through the equity

markets. . . . The talks could lead to expansion of joint marketing agreements, codevelopment of new business and clinical ventures or other cooperative arrangements short of a merger.[31]

Exploration of affiliations may result in canceling or postponing the idea, should research find that an alliance would be without value.

Negotiating an Alliance or Merger An organization should stay flexible. Flexibility may prompt the development of affiliations rather than mergers, or may lead to involvement in unexpected businesses, as more acceptable means of achieving expected outcomes. As the following example shows, the initial reasons for merging may lead to more business, based on practical reasons:

> PhyCor will assume the management of Straub Clinic and Hospital in Honolulu, which includes a 200 physician multispecialty group and a 159-bed hospital, under agreement reached in early October. . . . "It doesn't mean we're going into the hospital business: we're not," said Joseph Hutts, PhyCor's CEO. The finances and management of the 75-year-old clinic and hospital are so integrated that separating them would have been almost impossible. . . . Straub has a greater need for a capital partner than most multispecialty groups because it owns a hospital.[32]

Assessing the threat of operating agreements: Because full-asset mergers may not always work, some merger discussions become operating agreements for product- or business-specific purposes. Generally speaking, even tertiary affiliations pose threats to community providers when the operating agreement is accompanied by direct competition in the service area. An affiliation is not the same as a merger. The challenge to limited operating agreements is that continued competition by organizations in other areas of service always exits.

An example of competition among providers is the relationship between community and tertiary hospitals. With the proliferation of primary care practices placed in farther reaches of a referral area, expanded primary care networks created by both types of providers pose potential competitive threats. The same applies to payers who invest in physician practices in the market where they contract with established providers.

Choosing a limited affiliation: Program-specific affiliations, or limited affiliations, require the consideration of many scenarios in the event the other organization wishes to take action that adversely affects the other. In that case, the interests of one provider are negatively impacted by the intended actions of the other. However, if the tertiary provider found that specialty referrals were going to other tertiary providers, then the development of the primary care feeder sites is one way to secure the high-risk referral base initially sought in the service-specific affiliation.

An organization should develop memoranda of understanding reflecting the goals, followed by the final deal documents. Keeping the goals and focus of the alliance, operating agreement, or merger on track, is easily documented with a memorandum of understanding until the final documents are signed and approved. Such preliminary communication provides a set of working parameters to execute the arrangement, without getting lost in details that might detract from the overall purpose. The final deal documents will include financial, legal, and operational parameters.

Providing Support for the Alliance or Merger An organization wishing to enter into an alliance or merger should establish a team to manage and support the alliance. The group, consisting of representatives from all participating organizations, will oversee the creation of the alliance. In the case of a merger, transition teams sometimes work on specific issues, such as financial management, organizational structure, performance management systems, culture integration, and other important areas. The transition team may be a subcommittee reporting to an overseeing transition team or it may resolve all issues in one central committee. In the case of an alliance, management of the operating, financial, and market development activities may be performed by a management group within an existing structure. It is essential to share the activity among participating organizations and establish an infrastructure to manage it. Also, results should be monitored within a specific time frame in order to retain focus on the expected and actual purpose of the alliance.

Structuring the Acquisition Process Efficient collaboration requires financial and clinical incentives. The players should contribute to and participate in the extraordinary activities that direct the success of the merger or alliance, since they will also share the rewards of the integration. One system that moves actively to acquire other organizations structures its acquisition process in the following steps:

1. Align incentives.
2. Share ownership.
3. Share governance.
4. Avoid duplicative services.
5. Integrate management information systems strategy.
6. Contract globally.

Yet another organization explains the success of its operational strategy as dependent on the following components:

- vertical integration of all local medical services
- successful partnerships with physicians
- bottom-line management incentives
- significant upgrades of physical plants
- state-of-the-art information systems
- exclusive managed care contracts
- aggressive cost cutting

The lesson learned from these national firms is that in the long run any alliance or merger needs to be able to establish an attractive payer position and strong overall financial position to gain adequate revenues and market share.

Terms for dissolving an alliance: Even more important than the actual structure of the arrangement are the terms for dissolving the alliance, or termination provisions. These terms should include operating, financial, and change of ownership parameters. Examples of the types of thresholds that might be set up to trigger a notice period followed by a cure period and dissolution are

- time frame during which there are operating losses
- length of time for which the intended outcome is not working and for the divestiture process
- asset distribution, in the event there is a break up

CONCLUSION

Successful implementation of a strategic plan is truly a shared effort, and requires the input and effort of the entire organization. Management first reviews the plan and assigns accountability to various departments or individuals who will be responsible for key initiatives. Throughout implementation, management attention must be focused on the process, through continuous formal and informal update. Such updates should also extend to the entire organization; employees who are part of strategic changes and feel that their contributions are necessary to success will be able to innovate and experiment. Both the process and the results from enacting the strategy are important.

References

1. H. I. Ansoff and R. C. Brandenburg, "A Program of Research in Business Planning," *Management Science* XIII, no. 6 (1967): B219–B239.

2. "Strategic Planning: After a Decade of Gritty Downsizing, Big Thinkers Are Back in Corporate Vogue," *Business Week* (Aug. 22, 1996):

3. Mary K. Totten and others, *The Guide to Governance for Hospital Trustees* (Chicago: American Hospital Association, 1990), p. 4.

4. Peter Senge, *The Fifth Discipline: The Art and Science of the Learning Organization* (New York: Doubleday Currency, 1991).

5. Warren Bennis and Burt Nanus, *Leaders: The Strategies for Taking Charge* (New York: HarperPerennial, 1988), p. 206.

6. *Capitation Management Report 3,* no. 5 (May 1996): 65–71.

7. *Health Systems Review* (July/Aug. 1996): 24.

8. "Medical Transplants: Hospitals, Insurers Spend Tens of Millions to Acquire Physician Practices—and Gain Access to Patients," *Pittsburgh Business Times and Journal* 16, no. 39 (1997): 1.

9. *Fortune* 134 (Oct. 14, 1996): 82.

10. Adapted from *Medical Network Strategy Report* (July 1995): 8–12.

11. Adapted from Kristie Perry, "Would an MSO Make Your Life Easier?" *Medical Economics* (Apr. 10, 1995).

12. *Hospitals and Health Networks* (Aug. 5, 1995): 106.

13. William O. Cleverley, *The 1996–1997 Almanac of Hospital Financial and Operating Indicators* (Columbus, Ohio: Center for Healthcare Industry Performance Studies, 1996).

14. *Modern Healthcare* 26 (Sept. 30, 1996): 41.

15. *1996 Investment Management Institute Guide to Managing Financial Assets for Healthcare Systems, Hospitals, HMOs and Large Clinics* (Greenwich, Conn.: IMI, 1996), pp. 14–15.

16. *Hospitals and Health Networks* (Aug. 5, 1995): 102.

17. "IDFSs: Navigating through the Changing Currents," Erst & Young, L.L.P., 1996.

18. "Dynamics of Change: The Carle Clinic and Foundation Take a Leading Role in Managed Care while Continuing to Provide Traditional Fee-For-Service Medicine," *Health Care Review* (August 1996):

19. Interview with Dr. Richard Shea, vice president of medical affairs at Morton Plant Mease Health Care, St. Petersburg, Florida, Fall 1996.

20. William H. Davidow and Bro Uttal, *Total Customer Service: The Ultimate Weapon* (New York: Harper and Row, 1989), p. 109.

21. Presentation at SHSD&MD, American Hospital Association, September 1996.

22. Adapted from "Silver Lining," *AHA News* (June 17, 1996): 7.

23. *Modern Healthcare* 26 (Jan. 16, 1996): 17.

24. *Modern Healthcare* 26 (Aug. 5, 1996): 80.

25. *Modern Healthcare* 26 (Aug. 5, 1996): 88.

26. Deloitte and Touche's 6th biennial survey, "U.S. Hospitals and the Future of Health Care," summer 1996.

27. "NC Tax-Exempts Ponder Alliance," *Modern Healthcare* 26 (Sept. 9, 1996): 14.

28. "Partnership to Link NY, NJ Hospitals," *Modern Healthcare* 26 (Sept. 9, 1996): 16.

29. 1994 Columbia/HCA annual report.

30. *Modern Healthcare* 26 (Oct. 7, 1996): 8.

31. Ron Winslow, "Kaiser Permanente Unit, Group Health Enter Talks That Could Lead to Merger," *Wall Street Journal* (Aug. 16, 1996):

32. *Modern Healthcare* 26 (Oct. 7, 1996): 30.

6

Strategy as a Part of Organizational Life

The best laid plans of mice and men oft go astray.

—*Robert Burns*

Executive Summary

Upon emerging from an arduous strategic planning session, the return trip to the organizational life left behind can produce a shock. Organizations continue breathing, even as the future—promising or not—is being charted. For the between-cycle time, the establishment of strategic goals and the determination of new challenge is a dynamic process. It needs to be reviewed on a regular basis and made a formal component of the annual plan.

INTRODUCTION

Monitoring the corporate environment and communicating the relevant data forms one aspect of the strategic plan and sets the stage for further development. New alliances, new organizational structures, and new strategic directions make relationships different. New priorities and problems arise as a result of the implemented initiatives. The attention to strategic issues, apart from a formalized process, requires the same oversight structure used during the plan development and implementation process.

Between strategic plan developments, the organization needs to move in the direction of the vision. The activities involved in plan implementation are important components of strategy management. Management coordinates these activities and reports to the board. Involving the workforce in the strategic direction is critical to the implementation of a service delivery system. This chapter reviews the activities involved in organizational life in the period between planning cycles. It discusses how to manage progress of the plan and to evaluate the plan as it unfolds.

STRATEGIC PLAN REVIEW AND UPDATE

The strategic plan should be reviewed and updated annually. Specific objectives and activities are identified for completion as each division determines its strategic objectives. In *Vision in Action,* B. B. Tregoe discusses the case of a large life insurance company: "At the end of each fiscal year, each division manager reports his or her strategic plan to his or her superior. This includes action plans to implement it that are stated as critical issues. Last year's results in terms of critical issues resolved are also presented. This is done typically through detailed written reports. In addition, there are frequent informal, conversational checks at divisional and unit levels on the effectiveness of strategy implementation."[1]

The annual plan takes into account the current status and future outlook, but it also needs to be retrospective, by reporting on prior year performance compared to the stated goals and objectives. The challenges that arose in the implementation process also need to be addressed. The annual plan is the means of updating the strategy implementation schedule while allowing for contingencies, external changes, and internal repercussions based on these changes.

For example, many strategies in recent years have called for the creation of a primary care network to secure market share. The expected benefit of contracting in a closed-panel payer environment did not materialize, either with national reform or capitation growing out of the market. Further, hospitals were unfamiliar with these practices, and physicians rebelled against the lack of autonomy. Many hospitals acquired practices that had operating deficits, even before the acquisition costs were figured in. The choices were to cross-subsidize the practices, which would continue to operate at a loss; manage the process slowly over a course of five to seven years; make immediate and severe changes; or sell the practices privately in a partnership. With any of these choices, an effective strategic plan sets the pace.

The annual plan also must tie into the budget process. The financial forecasts and budgets are used to implement strategic initiatives and generate regular reports about what is or is not working. Volume, participation, cost, and revenue make up the plan review. Objective measures show whether the tactics are achieving expected outcomes. Leonard Goodstein has written, "The use of the budget to operationalize the strategic plan and the use of the budget review process as a constant measure of the organization's success in executing its strategic plan not only give life to the organization's budgeting processes, but also demand a strong commitment to the use of the budget on an ongoing basis."[2] Timing the annual planning process and the financial forecasting process so they are interdependent is critical to measuring progress and success.

The value of the annual strategic plan review comes in its ability to accomplish the following:

- identify the degree of integration
- determine whether the organization is responding to customer and community needs
- provide a framework for strategy monitoring
- provide meaningful updates to organization management
- implement an oversight structure for ongoing evaluation of the plan

Identify the Degree of Integration

Commitment to integration, on a full or partial basis, requires the same evaluation of the driving factors as any other full-scope commitment. Those driving factors that brought the organization to be committed to full or partial integration need to be assessed on an annual basis.

Changes in the Drivers for Integration Preparations for risk-shared reimbursement are under way for many providers. Providers not operating under capitation have little incentive to prepare for capitation if the area payers will not move in that direction. The evolution of managed care was expected to be resolved by integrated delivery systems (IDSs), but this expectation was based on continued growth in health care costs. Insurers, employers, and public programs such as Medicare and Medicaid have exhibited new levels of cost savings. Physician salaries stabilized in 1995, and the growth of medical expense as a percent of gross national product has slowed. One analyst has written: "Employers and consumers are asking the health care system for something very different: a seemingly incongruous mixture of broad choice and economic discipline. Employers and consumers are profoundly reluctant to disrupt long-standing relationships with physicians and hospitals that have met their needs in the past."[3]

It can be difficult to develop integration systems for purposes other than enhanced position with payers. In particular, the expense of acquisition and ongoing debt conflicts with the push to decrease costs. Types of integration other than full-asset integration are evolving, including what is known as virtual integration, where there is a range of alliances to be formed. These more modest models are becoming more popular in light of marketplace indicators that require fast price decreases, provider choice options, and access to new core competencies.

The reasons to pursue integration should be multiple, as any individual reason might not be as persuasive under changing market conditions. With single drivers for a strategy, there should be complete certainty for its completion. Nevertheless, one commentator quipped: "My experience to date with developing integrated delivery systems confirms the wisdom of the experienced financial forecasters: It will cost more to build than everybody predicted and it will make less money than everybody expected."[4]

Challenges to Integration Integration has its challenges. Alliances, mergers, and the formation of IDSs can be halted by the challenges of merging cultures and making decisions about assets and leadership. One account of a deal in a mid-sized Midwestern city describes how it

> fell apart over a proposal to consolidate acute care services in one of the two campuses. From a distance, the formula looked like a sure winner. A large tertiary care hospital downtown, where 90 percent of the specialists worked, would merge assets over a year or so with a smaller, less technology-heavy hospital in the suburbs, grab 50 percent market share and compete as a small system against the other hospital in town. But despite the overwhelming association between volume and quality in specialty services, despite the steady growth of managed care in the marketplace, despite the promise of the smaller hospital CEO sitting on top the new health system, the plan represented too much change for the small institution and it scotched the deal.[5]

In the deregulated market, there is no time, no future end-state of the industry to aspire to, and the providers' stability is often uncertain. There are contracts to be obtained, and payer accounts are changing rapidly in the current binge of acquisitions. In assessing an integration decision, the three practices help the decision maker to keep some perspective:

- Identify and assess the validity of driving forces behind the initial commitment to the goal.
- Identify and assess changes in payers and customers in the marketplace.
- Develop a list of options to pursue in light of actual and potential changes.

The development of tactics to support a strategic initiative hinges on understanding the instability of the market and the industry. With integration, groups and individuals that had previously been competitors have to get reacquainted as collaborators. They learn each other's lingo and read a common script in order to share a global review and avoid collisions.

Key Factors for Effective Integration   The deciding factors that lead
to a strategic position in the market are the same factors that create clinical and organizational excellence. Benchmarking and consolidation
determine the effectiveness of integrated systems.

Successfully using the benchmarking concept requires the participating organization (1) to identify processes for benchmarking and (2) to
identify like markets or organizations for comparison. Benchmarking has
been defined as "a continuous, systematic process for evaluating the
products, services, and work processes of organization that are recognized as representing best practices for the purpose of organizational
improvement."[6] Benchmarking requires a measurement that can be
recreated over time. The value of benchmarking is in understanding the
organization's position not only at a point in time but over time. Anything
from individual products and services to entire integration strategies can
be benchmarked.

To find like organizations or markets upon which to base comparisons, outside expertise can be called in. Many consulting firms provide
industry benchmark data, but they are distinguished by their philosophy of benchmarking. For example, one firm compares charges and
revenue per full-time equivalent (FTE) physician and operating costs
per FTE physician in systems without capitation and systems with high
capitation.[7]

Best practices can be found inside the health care industry, but they
can be found outside as well. For example, L. L. Bean is noted for its
excellent inventory management, and other companies that have sought
to perform with the same excellent standards have learned from them.
The Disney concept of service training is another notable extra-industry
performer.

The identification of best practices offers lessons for other providers.
The Health Care Financing Administration (HCFA) studied and cited managed care organizations in early 1997 for best practices and for excellence; their findings are given in table 6-1. The use of comparative
standards in IDSs actually enlarges the scope of performance measures
for managing success. Larger systems, such as the for-profit systems,
have a standard that is measured within their own system, and enhanced
efficiencies are a constant strategy.

The second key strategy for effective integration has to do with the
difficult decisions about resource allocation and combining services. It
can be challenging to move from the theoretical realm of strategizing to
the practical application of strategy. One of the more visible organizations facing these challenges is Columbia/HCA, whose operations are run
as a regional organization with several locations. The team focus for the
corporation means facing these challenging resource decisions on a regular basis: "This regional focus is often most visible when Columbia/HCA
eliminates duplicate services in neighboring facilities or in some cases

TABLE 6-1. Managed Care Organizations Cited by HCFA
for Best Practices

Organization	Distinction
Blue Cross and Blue Shield of Minnesota, St. Paul	Physician profiling, outcome measurement, utilization management
Blue Cross and Blue Shield of the Rochester (N.Y.) Area	Case management, case-mix severity adjustment
Cigna HealthCare of Arizona, Phoenix	Screening and prevention
Harvard Community Health Plan, Brookline, Mass.	Continuous quality improvement, physician profiling, outcomes measurement, technology assessment
Health America of Pittsburgh	Continuous quality improvement, protocol application
Health Partners, Minneapolis	Protocol applications, special population care coordination
Prudential Insurance Co., Roseland, N.H.	Technology assessment
United HealthCare Corp. Minneapolis	Performance measurement, provider communication utilization management

closes an entire facility. Decisions are made for the good of the region, where 'good' is defined primarily on the basis of bottom-line financial performance and meeting the needs of local customers (patients and physicians)."[8]

The staff pulls together and integrates according to a specified framework. One approach is to divide functional processes into three parts: planning, organization, and measurement and reporting. Such a framework calls for the following conditions:

- an authority and influence process that fosters collaborative decision making
- set of conflict resolutions processes that addresses the many kinds of conflict that can and will arise in the course of achieving clinical integration
- a motivation process that encourages managers and physicians to act in the best interest of the IDS overall
- a set of cultural maintenance activities that helps to create a common culture across the disparate entities that comprise the IDS.[9]

An efficient system maximizes existing services and eliminates duplicate services. As discussed in chapter 4, Crozer-Keystone consolidated their operations to form one single operational system management team, at which time they were able to appreciably improve the management of their services. The united management teams were better able to achieve results for the system, particularly after they revised the performance management systems to invest the leaders of the divisions in the system's rather than the division's performance. In Boston, the merger of Beth Israel Hospital and New England Deaconess Hospital also resulted in a more streamlined organization. Beth Israel Deaconess Medical Center has one management team and one set of clinical chiefs. The consolidated hospital is combining operations and retaining the strengths of the systems and the cultures.

In her *Market Driven Health Care,* Regina Herzlinger recommends a strategy analogous to virtual integration called focused factories (a term borrowed from the manufacturing sector). These structures provide convenient specialized care for victims of a certain chronic disease, or for those who need a particular form of surgery, or for those who require a diagnosis, checkup, or treatment for a routine problem. Under such a scenario, the providers and payers can develop relationships and contracts with relevant experts in each area.

Once consolidation is achieved, key decisions have to be made about what the system will look like. Consolidation with mergers and alliances make for hard decisions and closings. These decisions need to take place based on realistic expectations of utilization and demographics and on changing capabilities in technology and service delivery.

Health care organizations developing IDSs can employ physicians, but there's a catch: A physician practice acquisition is necessary to long-term survival, and comes with a significant risk to the acquiring organization. The Healthcare Financial Management and Physician Services of America surveyed 5,300 hospital chief financial officers about physician practice acquisition and reported the following findings:

- Only 17 percent have posted positive returns on their practice investments.
- Only 32 percent of acquired physician practices met revenue and expense projections set by the hospital.

According to an article in the *AMA News,* "Experts attribute these abysmal financial results to poor strategic planning by hospitals, low physician productivity, and executives' ignorance of practice management basics."[10]

The primary drivers of these results are that closed panel and capitated arrangements have not turned out as expected. This experience is partly what makes professional physician practice management firms (PPMs) so attractive. The arrangement whereby physicians invest in their future and maintain their autonomy and the firm provides management expertise and capital is appealing to hospitals, but by introducing a third party the benefits are automatically diminished.

Differences in culture and management styles and, perhaps, the disconnection in value and vision, impede physician practice management ventures by hospitals and integrated health care systems. The result can be a decision to divest. Notably, for-profit PPMs are growing from the divestment of HMOs and hospitals and have management expertise and access to capital behind them. Thirty publicly traded PPMs hold more than 30,000 physicians, about 5 percent of the nation's total.[11]

St. Joseph Medical Center in Towson, Maryland, demonstrates how a provider affiliation can yield payer contracting benefits. The provider affiliated without direct management responsibility for physician groups. The vice president of planning, marketing, and public relations explained:

> St. Joseph secured relationships through equity participation with groups of primary care providers, with the goal of ensuring access to the largest possible pool of service residents. In Maryland, rate review regulations have been inhibiting hospitals from negotiating capitated or discounted rates. Therefore, the primary care physicians have been channeling patients into the delivery system, while hospitals cannot use payer contracts to channel patients.
>
> Affiliations with strategically significant physician group practices were endeavored, including one with Doctors Health System, the first management service organization of an equity model physician group. As the first regional hospital to invest in an equity model physician group as a minority equity partner, St. Joseph Medical Center realized the following benefits:
> - St. Joseph Medical Center does not have to own physician practices to set the kind of goals that other organizations reach by requiring total control.
> - St. Joseph Medical Center can take on a major role in management care contracting and provider networking without controlling through acquisition or ownership.
> - St. Joseph Medical Center has developed primary care physician linkages that appeal to each segment of primary care physicians and thus successfully competes with other practice management options.[12]

Determine Whether the Organization Is Responding to Customer and Community Needs

Customer expectations change. The government has pulled back in its role of prescribing the parameters of health care delivery at the same time that baby boomers have become a more powerful force in decision making. The generation that grew up questioning authority now questions the care processes of clinicians. By taking an active interest in care, they are changing care systems and putting the patients—the customers, themselves—at the center. Regina Herzlinger writes, "The key to the successful transformation of the retailing, automobile, and information industries has been consumer supremacy . . . . Consumers vote with their dollars. . . . Responding to the needs of the consumer revolutionary requires a daring, visionary business person, not a bureaucrat or a social engineer."[13]

The variation in types of products and range of choice makes the customer the focal point for determining the how, when, and why of health care delivery. The customer propels strategic planning and annual planning. Some limits on consumer choices will continue to be valid until employers move to a voucher system that lets the employee completely decide the criteria in selecting payers, but as reported in *Hospital and Health Networks,* these limits are receding:

> Millions of health care consumers . . . want a new partnership, one in which patients bring information of their own to the table, to discuss their treatment options in detail and make informed, consensual decision. Many such judgments relate to personal values, lifestyle choices and calculation of health risks. . . . The old model of the doctor-patient relationship, in which doctors explained relatively little and patients did whatever they were told, is near dead. . . . In many cases, it is the doctors that are listening—really listening—to the patients.[14]

Obtaining Customer Opinions and Perceptions The changing shape of the delivery system in every marketplace requires a constant check on the opinions of those served. Reports of polls taken to gauge customer preferences show up with increasing frequency on the evening news, and those shaping the service delivery organizations take notice. Word-of-mouth recommendations and complaints about hospital experiences also have an impact on the public perception of an organization, but of course these tales are harder to monitor.

The trade association for hospital and health care networks commissioned market information on the perceptions of health care organizations. From May to September 1996, the American Hospital Association conducted a study on the status of public trust in the health care system. According to a summary published in *Modern Healthcare,* "The public backlash against hospitals is largely due to the perception that hospitals and other segments of the health care industry are more interested in making money than caring for patients." [15] The three components of this perception—"profit motivation," "waste out, quality in," and "losing legitimacy"—are elaborated in figure 6-1.

FIGURE 6-1. Consumer View on Hospitals

- *Profit motivation:* The public believes it understands the direction in which hospitals are moving—that hospitals are placing a priority on profit above a commitment to caring—but the public still isn't certain whether hospitals are acting of their own volition or largely as a consequence of the profit-driven mandates of health insurance companies or for-profit corporations.

- *Waste out, quality in:* The public doesn't understand the budgetary pressures that hospitals face. Consumers believe that if waste, fraud, and abuse were removed from health care, hospitals would be able to provide higher-quality care at more reasonable prices and still earn fair profits.

- *Losing legitimacy:* Hospitals are at risk of losing public support in maintaining their place at the table of health care decision making. As they lose the image of being "on the side" of the patient and making medical decisions based on what is best for the patient, they lose the public legitimacy to exercise the authority to which their expertise otherwise would entitle them.

Source: American Hospital Association.

Focusing on Measures of Quality and Satisfaction Focus has intensified on the Health Plan Employer Data and Information Set (HEDIS) database and the comparative measures of quality and satisfaction. The measures are primarily for employers and other public payers. For many large-scale purchasers and payers, the measure of satisfaction is the measure of quality. Although some managers do not trust nonclinicians to make judgments about clinical delivery, it is understood that the criteria on which users judge their care—access to care and relationship with the clinician—are paramount to a successful clinical care plan. Satisfaction ratings, therefore, can provide industry standards by which to measure organizations. Organizations take the opportunity to explore the best practices in the satisfaction arena. One consulting firm has calculated the cost of acquiring a new customer to be more than six times the cost of retaining an existing customer.[16] The financial value of keeping customers is very clear.

The HEDIS 3.0 version of measures provides comparative satisfaction scores given by participating payers. The presentation of these data has merit with the purchasers—both employers and public programs—and offers a market-driven opportunity to enhance the health care delivery system in ways that are concrete and meaningful to the customer. There are a variety of companies that provide satisfaction information. The NCQA has set standards for measuring patient satisfaction that are a required part of credentialing payers. Providers who conduct their own similar measurements (and subsequent initiatives) are well positioned in the competitive marketplace.

Health care organizations that are successful in the future will be ones that respond to customer needs. In the context of the planning cycle, that means continued attention to the customer and community needs. Changes in customer need equal changes in the marketplace.

Exploring Branding Strategies With the onset of acquisition of physician practices, hospitals transforming to health care delivery organizations appear substantively different to the consumer. Because of the transformation in most health care organizations in recent years and the changes expected in the years to come, packaging or branding is a way of enhancing customer relations. Helping customers identify new configurations of services and new organizational structures is part of demonstrating value to the customer base. The organization's definition of its internal culture and operations drives this branding strategy, as does the level of integration.

The growth of complex health care delivery systems brings with it a growth in branding efforts. The purpose of the branding is to concentrate a lot of concrete and abstract messages—including the organization's mission, vision, and values—into one symbol. The brand name's purpose is to create buyer confidence in the service and encourage repeated use of health care services. Business marketing practices rely on brands as a tool for attracting customers, bolstering reputation, and creating name recognition. Branding can fail, however, if the consumer benefits are not explicitly identified.

Brand development means not only creating customer-oriented value to differentiate one service from other services, but also maintaining the advantage. Harvard Business School's *Field Guide to Marketing* advises, "Nescafé and Kellogg have retained their market leadership because they have spent much of the premium in their prices on constantly developing new products and improving existing ones."[17] Successful branding is iterative and incremental and requires attention on at least an annual basis, as part of the planning process.

In addition, brand name should be applied with consistency for the service standards offered. One health system has developed service standards that must be enforced before any subsidiary organization takes on its name. Those service standards represent proven quality to users.

Some for-profit organizations have been able to grow or acquire businesses in multiple geographic areas and have sufficiently consolidated services to enable them to develop brand recognition for their services and products as part of a national campaign. The development of a central base of products, developed with a similar set of service standards, defines the brand and registers it in the minds of customers. For example, the goal of Columbia/HCA Healthcare is to make the name synonymous with health care, in the same way that Kleenex is synonymous with tissue. In July 1996, they established a national consumer call center that consolidates the physician referral centers from all their hospitals. Customer service representatives make referrals, schedule appointments, and provide other information. Columbia selects their representatives carefully and trains representatives for a period of three weeks. In a similar strategy, Manor Care, the nation's fourth-largest long-term care provider, made good on their goal of reaching adult children who live in different states than their parents: They acquired services in several more states and began identifying themselves as a nationwide provider.

National branding attracts national attention. As long as health care delivery continues to be regional and the markets are unique, regional branding efforts need to look to national successes, tailoring their message to a regional scale.

Provide a Framework for Strategy Monitoring

Because the strategic plan development process generates large volumes of information, ongoing communication is an integral part of the between-plan cycle. The organization keeps consumers or affiliated members in touch with its changes and innovations. Keeping the local and civic leadership informed should be part of networking and information meetings. The onset of community-oriented services has brought about or reinvigorated community advisory groups. These are helpful in interacting on common issues as well as keeping abreast of evolving needs and developments. The status of the annual and strategic plan can be appraised on a community level.

Strategic Plan Monitoring Strategic monitoring and providing relevant updates to the plan both complete one implementation and prepare for the development of the next plan. An audit of the plan reviews the tactics and updates the progress made on each of them. The information that provided the basis for the strategic conclusions should be assessed to see that it is still accurate. The results of environmental monitoring, which would likely already have been reported to the planning committee, need to be incorporated into the updated strategic plan at the time of the annual update.

Strategic management is partly strategic control of the process. While this function might be confused with implementation, the management agenda is the ongoing realization of the vision. Much of it has to do with resolving strategic directions and responding to new unintended stimuli.

Scenario Management The development of scenarios is a necessary component to managing the planning effort. This scenario management— monitoring the environment and making the relevant adaptations—is an effective means of tracking a complex industry in a complex environment. According to Peter Schwartz in *The Art of the Long View,* "Scenarios are a tool for helping us to take a long view in a world of great uncertainty. . . . Scenarios are stories about the way the world might turn out tomorrow, stories that can help us recognize and adapt to changing aspects of our present environment."[18] See figure 6-2 for the key steps in scenario development.

Identifying actions in scenario planning is more easily done if there are focal questions. It helps to look at the external environment with an eye to analyzing key decisions in that environment. Decisions have to be made about issues generated by the organization itself and about issues thrust upon the organization by the environment.

- Should we build a big ambulatory primary care medical practice in a suburb 10 miles away?
- Should we discontinue maternity services?
- Should we add an open heart surgery program?
- How should we respond to a hospital management or physician practice management firm buying a competitor?

List forces in the local environment that would affect success or failure in that decision:

- facts about customers, suppliers, competitors (from internal and external environment)
- trends in the macro environment: political, social, demographic, environmental, technological

Rank those driving factors by importance and uncertainty. Then plot the most important and most uncertain—those are the ones that call for the development of scenarios.

Scenario development is useful in looking at important issues where the future is uncertain. Fleshing out those scenarios identifies potential implementation strategies. All of the implications, positive and negative, need to

FIGURE 6-2. Key Steps to Scenario Development

1. Identify focal issue or decision
2. Identify key forces in the local environment
3. Identify the driving forces
4. Rank by importance and uncertainty
5. Select scenario logic
6. Flesh out scenarios
7. Identify implications
8. Identify leading indicators and signposts

Source: Peter Schwartz, *The Art of the Long View* (New York: Doubleday/Currency, 1991).

be explored. That means basing research on both objective data collection and subjective viewpoints. The more factors taken into consideration, the more useful the anticipation. There are three basic scenarios that make different assumptions about how the environment will change:

1. *More of the same, but better:* This scenario anticipates growth in both the economy and in the industry. This is the type of scenario that occurred after World War II, amid economic growth and the expectation that government would provide medical services.
2. *Worse:* This one suggests that the economy will enter a period of slow growth or a recession and that the industry will suffer. The 1970s saw inflation in the price of natural resources, which brought about an awareness of the crisis in health care costs. The industry moved toward cost management and cost reduction.
3. *Different but better:* The economy shifts, and the industry experiences a fundamental social change. In recent years, when capitation was expected to take hold throughout the industry, nobody knew what to expect. But the health care industry has revitalized its commitment to wellness and to injury and illness prevention, with the development of policies and practices that promote healthy living.

Scenario management can also look to more macro forces shaping the industry. Of the following trend categories, only a few clearly have direct relevance to what is happening in the health care industry. Nevertheless, as Michael E. Porter argues in his *Competitive Strategy,* factors on the periphery of the industry can exert a vast influence.[19] These seemingly peripheral factors may represent the future in the minds of consumers:

- *Technology:* Most management textbooks in the last decade deal with information technology and how it will change society. As are companies in every industry, health care organizations are investing large amounts of financial and human resources in keeping up with information revolution.
- *Politics:* The history of health care in recent years could not be written without referring to rising costs and the maldistribution of physicians. Newspaper and television stories on patients who fall through the cracks of managed care shape the directions and expectations for health care organizations.
- *The self-help movement:* The onset of the self-help movement is a prelude to the growing popularity of alternative medicine. In the holistic approach to the culture, such factors as new age music, alternative medicine, and health foods all relate to the health care setting.
- *Cottage industries:* Microbreweries and independent manufacturers of all kinds represent the reverse of contemporary trends that

show massive companies diversifying into every industry, but such cottage industries may represent a future for those who still expect courteous and personal attention.

The monitoring process requires an open mind. It requires one to suspend disbelief, because you never know what may signal changes in the marketplace, changes in the industry, and changes for the organization. It calls for the conviction that anything could happen. Peter Schwartz cites the example of Hollywood and the videocassette recorder: "[Hollywood] saw it as a threat throughout the 1970s and the 1980s. Even at the Academy Award ceremonies, stars decried the loss of the 'silver screen experience' as a means of enjoying movies, compared to watching videos at home. They didn't see that suddenly there would be enormous new revenues. They didn't ask, 'What if it doesn't kill the theater business?' They considered only the scenario in which the VCR destroyed them. . . . They fought the VCR hard and delayed it successfully and lost millions of dollars in the process."[20]

The warning signals or signposts along the way that point to industry changes are ones to watch. In figuring out the right signals, it is important not to let emotions and worries get in the way and to pick signals that are specific enough. Schwartz notes that demographers in the early 1990s had the following experience with the maternity marketplace:

American demographers failed to predict the "echo baby boom"—the massive increase of births [in the 1980s] among women aged 35 to 45. The demographers could have easily avoided the embarrassment (for them) and expense (for local governments) by asking themselves, "What factors might indicate a change in the large trend?" They might have noticed a small emerging industry for in vitro fertilization in the early 1980s. Its mere existence would suggest that older women could have babies in greater numbers. If its popularity soared as those women began to run up against their biological clocks, that would suggest that more older women would want to have babies."[21]

Scenario management calls for continually updating the data supporting the strategic inputs in the environment, as well as watching larger trends in and out of the industry. Such attention may lead the organization in a direction that is broader than health care delivery and will help to chart the future and to find the path to achievement of the vision.

Provide Meaningful Updates to Organization Management

Every action has a reaction. For any action taken by a health care organization, the responses of the customers and other providers may in turn influence the direction of the organization. The form and content of meaningful updates in industry trends must be sensitive to continued shifts and amenable to revision. The priorities on the managerial agenda require constant attention.

Implement an Oversight Structure for Ongoing Evaluation of the Plan

The structure for evaluation may be set up so that the plan's development can easily be reviewed and reexamined for continued reliance on the assumptions in the plan. The plan identified directions. Acting on such directions as cost efficiency and market penetration, the evaluation process can result in modifications to the guiding spirit of the strategic planning process.

The planning evaluation has the following components:

- review process
- intervening variables
- course correction and modification
- planning committee updating and education

The vision, the environmental data, internal assessment, key issues, conclusions, and strategic directions are all evaluated as part of this process.

Review Process   The review process is for examining the plan's components, inherent assumptions, available information, and the subsequent planned outcomes and deviations in the implementation process. The process helps to determine the extent to which the variances were based on new information. The review process keeps the plan an active part of the organization. The process has seven steps:

1. *Measure the continued relevance of the issues identified in the plan:* In the event that during the implementation process, other priorities take over the management team's agenda, then it is time to review how the plan prioritizes issues. If issues are no longer relevant, and have not been dealt with during the implementation process, this is the time to take them off the agenda.
2. *Evaluate the analytical framework of the strategy and tactics:* The information that was available at the time of the planning process may have been updated, or projections may not have become realities. The basis of the strategy may have been founded on data that turned out to be less important than other data.
3. *Correct the course:* The course correction, based on new information or an effective change of priorities, may occur naturally as

the implementation proceeds, but a comprehensive review is a good time to reestablish priorities. The health care organization's priorities may be adjusted to address external and internal factors that bring about changes: new modalities of care, differing payer allowances, and the threat of health care reform.

4. *Review the plan with any new leadership:* That includes the board, medical staff, and management. New board chairs, new CEOs, and new medical staff presidents often come with operating priorities left over from their earlier experiences. Although their experience and expertise can influence to the overall direction, the emphasis should be on building a consensus.

5. *Modify service delivery plans:* Given specific financial and operational criteria, management teams review services and new programs to decide their direction based on actual performance compared with projected performance and overall viability. Health care providers resist the closure of services that have no market, differentiating value to potential customers, or financial viability, but projects that are not meeting projections, once given enough time to break even or to reach goals, become a drain on resources that could be used elsewhere. A structure for determining when to let a project go was developed by Jennings, Ryan & Kolb for the Society for Healthcare Planning and Marketing. (See figure 6-3.)

- *Evaluate the stakeholders:* Evaluate the stakeholders in the planning process and the level of change in their priorities. This evaluation also includes the planning process based on input from potential customers of the health care organization, the proper professional leadership, the responsibilities of the management

FIGURE 6-3. Criteria for Evaluating Projects

- Is the actual financial performance comparable to the anticipated financial performance?
- Is there a comparable service of similar size to justify its current situation?
- Is there a reason for lower utilization and future projections accordingly?
- Is the actual payer mix comparable to the anticipated payer mix?
- Is the level of fixed cost relative to expansion?
- Can the spin-off benefits be quantified to the overall health care organization or system?
- Is the service differentiated from competitors?
- Are there action steps to reverse losses that can be taken?
- Is this a mature service?
- Would you invest your paycheck in this service?

Source: Jennings, Ryan & Kolb, "Measuring the Results of the Strategic Plan." Annual Meeting of the Society for Healthcare Planning and Marketing, spring 1991.

team, along with the options available through the guidance of the board of trustees and the medical staff's clinical leadership. The issues to raise would include an analysis of stakeholder response pre- and postimplementation.

- *Review major services:* Serious review requires reevaluation of major services relative to prior plan assumptions, including budget impact and incremental patient volume expectations. Reevaluation should cover progress toward identified goals, operating performance in strategic areas, review of response to intervening variables, and assessment of the process used to obtain the actual results.

The progress toward goals is likely the product of the plan that outlined specific tasks and activities for management to undertake. A comparison of the project list from the strategic plan is comprehensively reviewed with the management team during the implementation phase. Variations from the intended action plan are noted with the purpose of assessing the accuracy, timeliness, and feasibility of the plan.

Intervening Variables "Intervening variables" are changes in the environment since the plan was developed. They can take the form of new information or new developments. The introduction of new services in the marketplace or the closure of old ones must be accounted for. Acute care providers may change their scope of services, leaving a gap in or creating additional demand on the organization. New entrants into the health care provider marketplace are also a consideration, for example, insurers purchasing physician practices in order to increase their own market share. (Instances of such strategies can be found in other industries: Hershey's bought Friendly's in order to control its own distribution, and PepsiCo used the strategy of purchasing fast food franchises, such as Taco Bell, in order to increase the sales of its products.) These new entrants into the service provider business start to compete with the hospital for relationships with admitting physicians. They compete for the control of physicians for direct admissions and for specialty referrals.

Some demographic changes can affect the types of medical care the market demands. For example, increased urban problems can result in a middle class migration to the suburbs, leaving a higher than expected number of rented and vacant homes. There are significant differences in the medical needs of the middle-class population, many of who are homeowners, and those who live at or below the poverty level, most of who are renters.

Insurers or direct employers may make changes in their health care provider relationships or payment schemes that deliberately or inadvertently bring about changes for the health care organization. For the provider that has a short-term notice in the contract, payers may termi-nate contracts in order to bring about more financially advantageous terms, creating hardships for the health care organizations. Contract terms and duration must be reviewed with an eye on risk.

An employer, forced to make changes to respond to an increase in costs, may take an insurer that has no relationships with a local provider, or an insurer in the midst of negotiations that never amount to anything. In either case, the employer has made a decision to lower cost, often to the detriment of the provider. In a environment crowded with providers, the employer may have taken the risk of consolidating the health care services at one of the providers in return for a savings. Such a move by an employer has repercussions for the provider that may not have been foreseen at the development of the plan.

New regulations at a national and statewide level that affect service delivery and reimbursement can create a shortfall that has to be man-aged directly or managed with adjustments to services or financial plans. A carefully planned management agenda remains flexible.

Course Correction and Modification "Course correction" is the response to new variables that change the plan, either new information or developments discovered in the implementation and evaluation process. With the variety of information emerging from the review process, the evaluation should consist of three components:

1. For what we knew, how did we do?
2. For what we didn't know, how did we do?
3. For what we now know, what will we do next?

Once things happen, it's a whole new place, or a whole new system, or whole new organization.

Finally, the vision and strategic direction should be reassessed in light of the update. If they require modification, it is better to make the adjust-ments before embarking on a multiyear process than to have no clear out-comes or expected value. As the vision and values are revisited annually, so are the range of action items that set the pace for the year to come. The strategic plan accounts for the new organization and the new environment.

Planning Committee Updating and Education Report the strategic plan status and continue planning committee education on relevant top-ics. The planning committee should be formally apprised of the progress on the strategic agenda, and it needs to reaffirm its commitment to the vision and values articulated in the plan. The focus of the educational component is achievement of the vision.

The year after completion of the strategic plan, regular meetings of the planning committee address the strategic plan and operational issues. Topics for this meeting can include the following:

- relevant external information and implications for the organization
- relevant internal information and implications for the organization
- progress to date on completed initiatives and their results
- next year's anticipated initiatives

In successive years, the organization will conclude initiatives, revise the strategic plan, and process new environmental information. The planning committee needs to meet regularly, including an annual meeting to review the strategies in progress.

The pace of change in health care delivery and payment has accelerated dramatically in the last few years, and regular extensive discussion of new events is worthwhile. Briefings of the planning committee, and possibly the entire board as well, can focus on areas of the strategic plan that are affected by rapid industry change. Topics should be those that management determines are the "hottest," areas of care delivery that are facing the greatest change. In the last few years, most health care delivery organizations have been wrestling with physician practice development, managed care contracting, and institutional relationships. All of the foregoing potentially reshape the directions of the organization, and even if an organization has decided not to engage in any of the new arrangements, it is useful to review the thought process behind those decisions.

The annual comprehensive meeting of the planning committee and the board subtly reaffirms the investment in and commitment to the vision. As long as the vision continues to make sense, there is no need to create a new strategic plan.

The planning committee would have seen information through the year at their meetings as new market information and organizational performance reports become available. Specifically, the ongoing updates (or those that are candidates for presentation at an annual update) include the following:

- recent market share information
- recent market research from consumers and purchasers
- recent operating performance indicators
- updates on market-based payers and providers
- updates on local service delivery collaboration
- updates on the physician network
- status on regional collaboration through merger/alliance options
- revised assumptions from the plan and a revised action plan
- revised profit-and-loss statement
- scenario updates

The attention to strategic issues has a different process but uses the same oversight structure used during the plan development and implementation process. The process includes the following exchanges of information:

- report to the planning committee and the board during the time frame between strategic plans
- presentation of annual plans and the key budget assumptions and the progress made on the plan to date
- review of all key initiatives and their status with the planning committee
- report to the planning committee about organizational performance relative to the annual plans on at least a quarterly basis, relative to the system's volumes
- review of the initiatives in the context of the strategic plan and the annual plan
- review of the vision statement and affirmation of the continued commitment to the vision statement and the strategic directions

Planning sessions to review and establish a future framework may take place during two-day retreats or over multiple meetings lasting several hours each. The newer the organization and planning committee are to strategic planning, the lengthier the presentation to acquaint them with an analytic context for decision making and the broad range of issues to manage. The agenda's content (the amount of information to be presented to the planning committee) and the work to be done in the committee meetings determine the time needed for the process. It is up to management to decide whether to provide summary analyses or detailed information.

The agenda is determined by what the planning committee knows already and how much has yet to be reviewed and discussed. The presentations also function as an educational forum and acquaint the committee members with the broad range of issues. The content of the meetings determines the frequency and content of the meetings. The standing planning committee would need less education in a strategic planning process, because the members are familiar with the organization's position and relevant issues.

The committee that meets regularly and reviews information about both the organization's performance and the marketplace requires less education about the marketplace than the committee that does not regularly review organization or market updates. The committee that is more current on strategic issues needs less outside expertise—such as a speaker on health care trends in another market or nationally, a summary on key issues affecting the organization or market, and a recommended strategy.

The scope of information reviewed with the committee depends on how recently and how extensively the committee has been briefed. If the committee is largely the same group as the year before, then the group does not need to have the details repeated to them. The individuals who are new on the committee can be updated in a small group meeting or in individual meetings with management. Table 6-2 reviews the level of information

TABLE 6-2. Scope of Strategic Issues Presentation

Recentness of the Last Update		
Up to a year ago	1–2.5 years ago	More than 2.5 years ago
Depth of Update		
Minimal	Moderate	Comprehensive
Issues to Present		
External update on focused market factors	External update on competitors and collaborators, changes in reimbursements, customer demands	Full strategy plan development
Strategy implementation	Strategy implementation update	Industry trends
Organizational performance	Organizational performance	Strategic assessment

related to how recently a presentation was made and makes recommendations of the scope of the update needed for the planning committee.

CONCLUSION

The organization thrives on its strategy. Review and update of the strategic plan help to keep it viable and relevant. Shifts in the field may call for adjustments, and shifts in consumer expectations demand a swift response. Responding to customer needs is a hallmark of the successful health care organization. Two of the tools for being prepared, scenario development and a thorough review process, keep the strategy an active part of organizational life.

References

1. B. B. Tregoe and others, *Vision in Action: Putting a Winning Strategy to Work* (New York: Simon & Schuster, 1989).

2. Leonard D. Goodstein, Timothy M. Nolan, and William J. Pfeiffer, *Applied Strategic Planning* (San Diego: Pfeiffer, 1992), p. 341.

3. Jeff Goldsmith, "Managed Care Mythology Supply Side Dreams Die Hard," *Healthcare Forum Journal* (Nov./Dec. 1996): 42-47..

4. J. Daniel Beckham, "The IDS as Moving Target," *Healthcare Forum Journal* (Sept./Oct. 96): 54.

5. Craig Havighurst and Anne Berdahl, "Health Systems Review," *Dispatch* (July/Aug. 1996): 8.

6. Michael J. Spendolini, *The Benchmarking Book* (New York: American Management Association, 1992), p. 9.

7. Medical Group Management Association, Englewood, Colo.

8. *Columbia/HCA: A National Profile,* p. 40.

9. David W. Young and Diana Barrett, "Managing Clinical Integration in Integrated Delivery Systems: A Framework for Action" *Hospital and Health Services Administration* 42, no. 2 (Summer 1997): pp. 255-79.

10. "Practices Sell, Hospitals Lose," *AMA News* (Dec. 11, 1995).

11. Mary Chris Jaklevic, "Practicing for Wall Street," *Modern Healthcare* (Jan. 6, 1997): 48.

12. Regina Herzlinger, *Market Driven Health Care* (Reading, Mass.: Addison-Wesley, 1997), p. 15.

13. Mark Hagland, "Power to the Patient," *Hospital and Health Networks* (Oct. 20, 1996): 25-30.

14. Charlotte Snow, "A Loss of Confidence," *Modern Healthcare* (Jan. 13, 1997): 3.

15. Presentation by Sachs, Healthcare Strategy Institute, Chicago (Apr. 30, 1996).

16. Jeffrey J. Lefko, interview by author, Towson, Maryland, 16 July 1997.

17. *Field Guide to Marketing* (Cambridge, Mass.: Harvard Business School Press, 1994), p. 5.

18. Peter Schwartz, *The Art of the Long View* (New York: Doubleday/Currency, 1991), p. 3.

19. Michael E. Porter, *Competitive Strategy* (New York: The Free Press, 1980).

20. Schwartz, *Art of the Long View,* p. 204.

21. Ibid., p. 209.

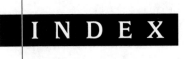

INDEX

Ability, 123–28
Accountability
    defining terms of, 137–38
    designating, 136–38
Acquisition process, structuring, 179–80
Activation, 119–23
Aetna Health Plans, 23
Affiliated medical practice corporation
        (AMPC), 95
Affiliations, 104–5, 172–73
    identifying added value of, 105–6
    understanding goals of, 105
Agenda, preparing, for planning process,
        38–41
Alliances
    creation of, 171–80
    negotiating, 178–79
    providing support for, 179
    strategic considerations for pursuing,
        174–75
    structure of, 175, 177–78
    terms for dissolving, 180
American Society for Healthcare Marketing
        and Public Relations, 21
American Society for Hospital Public
        Relations, 21
Analysis paralysis, 132
Area-adjusted per-capita cost (AAPCC) rates, 7
Articulation, 112–19

Biotechnology, 73
Branding strategies, 192–93
Buyer power, existing industry players, 84
Buyers Health Care Action Group, 58

Capitation, 2–3, 10, 11
    government-enacted, 9
    increased attention to, 60–61
Centralized presentations, 114
Cigna, 23
Cleveland Clinic, 5
Clinical activity and performance assess-
        ment, 92
Clinical practice guidelines as industry driver,
        73

Clinical treatment as industry driver, 73
Clinton Administration health care reform,
        11, 22
Collaborative marketing, 167–80
Columbia/HCA, 5, 8, 23
Commitment, lack of, 62–63
Committee agenda, developing, 40–41
Communication, effective, 116
Community, strategic plan and organiza-
        tional commitment to, 11–12
Community benefit and collaboration,
        169–70
Community Health Centers of Two Harbors,
        Minnesota, 15, 16, 17
Community health status, mistakes in, 107–8
Competitor forces, framework for assessing,
        81–85
Comprehensive Health Planning and Public
        Health Service Amendment Act
        (1966), 17
Conduct values clarification, 43–44
Consolidations, 172–73
Contract assessment, 94
Contract buyer assessment, 94
Contracting vehicle, developing, with or
        among physicians, 147–48
Cooley Dickenson Hospital, 173
Corporate restructuring, 20
Course correction and modification,
        200–201
Crozer-Keystone Health System, 118, 127
Customer groups, 100
    assessing, 101–2
    building databases on, 100–101
Customers
    getting and keeping, 57–61
    needs of, 99–102
    obtaining opinions and perceptions of,
        190–91
    satisfaction of, 59, 60

Dartmouth Atlas of Health Care, 7
Decentralized work groups, establishment of,
        119
Demographics as industry driver, 71–72

Departmental presentations, 115
Direct contracting, perceived advantages of, 75
Diversification, 20, 21

Economics as industry driver, 71
Employee alignment
    lack of, 63–65
    teams as tools for, 122
Employees
    establishing structures that support participation of, 117–18
    getting invested, 131
    guiding, through change, 130
Environmental analysis, 41–43
    lessons learned from performing, 106–8
Environment assessment, 69–108
    approach to affiliation, 104–6
    frameworks for health care industry
        delivery models, 89–91
        geographic, 102–4
        industry arena identification, 86–89
        internal organizational, 91–96
        market position, 96–102
        national trends, 85–86
    identifying industry drivers, 70–71
        clinical practice guidelines, 73
        clinical treatment, 73
        demographics, 71–72
        economics, 71
        finance and payment mechanisms, 74–75
        human resources, 72–73
        regulatory and political activities, 74
        technology, 73–74
    models for performing industry analysis, 78–85
    payer/provider landscape, 75–78
Equicor, 23
Equitable Life Assurance Society, 23
Ethical Foundation of New System Working Group, 11

Federal utilization review program, 18
Fee-for-service market, 60
Finance and payment mechanisms as industry driver, 74–75
Financial capability, current and potential, 55–56
Financial position assessment, 93
Flexibility, requirements for, 120
For-profit management firms for hospitals and physician practices, 4
For-profit providers, growth of, 23–24
Future statements, relating vision to, 45–46

Governance oversight, 120–21
Government-enacted capitation, 9
Graduate Medical Education National Advisory Committee (GMENAC), 16–17

Great Depression, 13
Great Society programs, 16
Gross national product (GNP), health care in, 3
Group Health Associates (GHA), 150–51
Group Health Cooperative of Puget Sound, 23

Health care delivery
    current state of, 2–3
    standardization of, 53–54
    trends in planning, 1–30
Health care delivery system
    heavy regulation in, 12–13
    models for, 89–91
Health Care Financing Administration (HCFA), 7, 71–72
Health care industry, growth of, 13
Health care network structures, changes in, 9
Health care service delivery, planning's role in development of, 12–24
Health care spending, increase in, 3
Health Maintenance Act (1973), 19
HealthPartners, 58
Health Plan Employer Data and Information Set (HEDIS), 7, 8, 24, 53, 191–92
HealthSouth, 24
Hill-Burton program, 15, 18
Historical statements, relating vision to, 45
Horizontal integration, 20
Hospital Corporation of America, 18
Hospital-focused organizations, evolution of, 123–24
Hospital Survey and Construction Act (1946), 14, 15
Human resources as industry driver, 72–73

Immunotherapy, 73
Independent practice association (IPA), 95
Industry analysis, models for performing, 75–85
Industry arena identification, 86–89
Industry components of service delivery system, 87
Industry drivers, identifying, 70–71
Industry players
    existing, 84, 85
    potential, 82–83, 83–84
Integrated delivery and financing systems (IDFS), 3
Integrated delivery systems (IDSs), 3
Integration
    challenges to, 186
    changes in drivers for, 185–86
    identifying degree of, 185–90
    key factors for effective, 187–90
    mistakes in, 107
Internal newsletters and updates, 114
Internal organizational assessment, 91–96
Intervening variables, 199–200

Joint Commission for the Accreditation of Healthcare Organizations, 53

Kaiser Health Plan, 15
Kaiser Permanente, 170

Labor Health Institute of St. Louis, 15
Lahey-Hitchcock Medical System, 173
Leaders, finding new, 130–31
Leadership, preparing, for planning process, 38–39
LifeSpan, 5

Managed care
  as factor in integration of health care delivery, 2
  growth of, 23
  movement toward more, 143–67
  prepaid, 74
  variation in penetration, 8–9
Management, commitment from, 119–20
Management services organization (MSO), 95
Management support, obtaining top-level, 137
Market assessments, 59
Market forces, 82
Marketing, 167–71
Market position assessment, 96–102
Market research, 59
Market share, 98–99
MedCath, 24
Medicaid, 17, 74
  shift of, to prepaid managed care programs, 2
Medicare, 17, 74
  shift of, to prepaid managed care programs, 2
Merger
  and alliance position, 56–57
  negotiating, 178–79
  providing support for, 179
Meridia Health System, 5
MetLife Healthcare, 23
MetraHealth Company, 23
Miner's Clinics, 15
Morristown (New Jersey) Memorial Hospital, 150

National Committee for Quality Assurance (NCQA), 7–8, 53
National Health Planning and Resources Development Act (1974), 17
National Medical Enterprise, 23
Nationwide service area, 104
NCQA, 7, 8, 24, 53, 55, 60
New England Medical Center (NEMC), 5
Nixon, Richard M., 16, 19

Organization
  articulating values of, 44
  financial capabilities, 160–67
  identifying values of, 43–44
  performance and capability of, 53–55

providing meaningful updates to management of, 197
response of, to customer and community needs, 190–93
strategy as part of life of, 183–203
OrNda, 23
Outsourcing, skill acquisition through, 127–28
Oversight structure, implementing, for ongoing evaluation of plan, 197–203

Participants, preparing, for planning process, 39–40
Payers, 168
  assessment and position of, 48–51
  establishing platform of, 144–47
  merging roles of, 25–29
  mistakes in relationships of, 107
  monitoring trends of, 150–51
  position assessment of, 93–96
Payment, preparing for changing modes of, 148–49
Performance management restructuring, 118–19
Performance measurement systems, 129–30
Phoenix Baptist Hospital and Medical Center, 150
PhyCor, 5, 8, 178
Physician assessment, 92
Physician bonding, 51–52
Physician-hospital organization (PHO), 95
Physician network assessment and position, 51–53
Physician network development, 151–60
Physician practice management firms, 153–58
Physician preference assessment, 94–95
Physicians, developing contracting vehicle with or among, 147–48
Physicians Quality Care, 8
Plan, definition of, 33
Plan development chart, 36
Planning. See also Strategic plan
  definition of, 1–2, 33
  role in development of health care service delivery, 12–24
  as tool for being prepared, 3–6
Planning committee updating and education, 201–3
PMH Health Services Network, 170
Polio epidemic, 13
Population characteristics, 97–98
Prepaid managed care system, 74
Presbyterian Hospital, 173
Primary care provider-specialist mix, 96
Primary service area, 102–3
Private health insurance market, 75
Promotion, 171
Providers
  changes in relationships of, 9–10

(continued on next page)

Providers *(continued)*
  merging roles of, 25–29
  shift in economic incentives for, 10
Prudential, 23

Quality indicator categories, 53
Quality of service delivery, 21

Reality testing, 132
Regional Health System Areas (HSAs), 17–18
Regulatory and political activities as industry
    driver, 74
Reporting structure, defining, 137
Revenue and market share considerations,
    173
Review process, 197–99

Sachs Group, 89
Salem (Oregon) Hospital, 150
Scenario management, 194–97
Secondary service area, 103–4
Selective contracting, 101
Senior management strategy meetings, pur-
    pose of, 138–39
Service array, 168–69
Service delivery system, industry compo-
    nents of, 87
Service directory, scope of, 87, 89
Skill acquisition, through outsourcing,
    127–28
Skill-specific training, 125–26
Social Security Amendment (1972), 19
Society for Healthcare Planning and
    Marketing, 21
Society for Healthcare Strategy and Market
    Development, 21
Society for Hospital Planning, 18–19
Staff training, 124–26
State Health Planning and Development
    Agencies (SHPDAs), 17
Statewide service area, 104
Strategic plan. *See also* Planning
  auditing prior, 35
  components of, 34
  development process, 33–66
  integrating organization's directions into,
    6–12
  monitoring, 193–94
  and organizational commitment to com-
    munity, 11–12
  and organization's vision and values,
    10–11
  review and update, 184–203
Strategic plan development
  definition of, 34
  past problems with, 62–66
  steps in process of, 34–62
    articulating vision statement, 45–47

clarifying organization's options, 47–61
conduct values clarification, 43–44
developing action plan, 61–62
environmental analysis, 41–43
preparing agenda for, 38–41
review prior plans and planning
    processes, 35, 37–38
Strategic plan implementation, 111–32
  ability, 123–28
  action steps in, 135–80
    designating accountability, 136–38
    focusing management attention,
      138–40
    moving organization toward change,
      142
    moving toward managed care and inte-
      gration, 143–67
    reporting on progress, 140–42
    rewarding change and experimenta-
      tion, 143
  activation, 119–23
  articulation, 112–19
  past problems with, 128–32
Strategy
  as part of organizational life, 183–203
  structure and agenda of meetings, 139–40
  translating, into action, 131–32
Strategy direction, communicating drivers
    for, 113–14
Substitute, threat of, 83–84
Supplier power, existing industry players, 85
SWOT analysis, 78–81

Tax Equity and Fiscal Responsibility Act
    (1982), 20
Teams
  creation of, 121–22
  diversity within, 122
  examples of successful, 122–23
  as tools for employee alignment, 122
  training of, 126–27
Technology as industry driver, 73–74
Tenet Healthcare, 5, 8, 23
Training, 124–27
Truman, Harry S, 14

Unions as force in developing prepaid group
    practices, 15
United HealthCare Corp. Aetna, 23
US Healthcare, 23

Value audit, conducting, 44
Vencor, 24
Vertical integration, 20
Vision, 45–46
Vision statement, developing, 46–47

War on Poverty, 17